Clinical Pathology

Editor

GEZA S. BODOR

CLINICS IN LABORATORY MEDICINE

www.labmed.theclinics.com

Editor-in-Chief
MILENKO JOVAN TANASIJEVIC

September 2018 • Volume 38 • Number 3

ELSEVIER

1600 John F. Kennedy Boulevard • Suite 1800 • Philadelphia, Pennsylvania, 19103-2899

http://www.theclinics.com

CLINICS IN LABORATORY MEDICINE Volume 38, Number 3
September 2018 ISSN 0272-2712, ISBN-13: 978-0-323-64103-6

Editor: Stacy Eastman
Developmental Editor: Laura Fisher

Reprints. For copies of 100 or more, of articles in this publication, please contact the Commercial Reprints Department, Elsevier Inc., 360 Park Avenue South, New York, New York 10010-1710. Tel. 212-633-3874, Fax: 212-633-3820, E-mail: reprints@elsevier.com.

Clinics in Laboratory Medicine (ISSN 0272-2712) is published quarterly by Elsevier Inc., 360 Park Avenue South, New York, NY 10010-1710. Months of issue are March, June, September, and December. Business and Editorial offices: 1600 John F. Kennedy Blvd., Suite 1800, Philadelphia, PA 19103-2899. Periodicals postage paid at NewYork, NY and additional mailing offices. Subscription prices are $263.00 per year (US individuals), $507.00 per year (US institutions), $100.00 per year (US students), $347.00 per year (Canadian individuals), $617.00 per year (Canadian institutions), $185.00 per year (Canadian students), $402.00 per year (international individuals), $617.00 per year (international institutions), $185.00 (international students). Foreign air speed delivery is included in all Clinics subscription prices. All prices are subject to change without notice. POSTMASTER: Send address changes to *Clinics in Laboratory Medicine*, Elsevier Health Sciences Division, Subscription Customer Service, 3251 Riverport Lane, Maryland Heights, MO 63043. **Customer Service: 1-800-654-2452 (US). From outside of the US and Canada, call 1-314-447-8871. Fax: 1-314-447-8029. E-mail: journalscustomerservice-usa@elsevier.com (for print support) or journalsonlinesupport-usa@elsevier.com (for online support).**

Clinics in Laboratory Medicine is covered in *EMBASE/Exerpta Medica, MEDLINE/PubMed (Index Medicus), Cinahl, Current Contents/Clinical Medicine, BIOSIS and ISI/BIOMED.*

Contributors

EDITOR-IN-CHIEF

MILENKO JOVAN TANASIJEVIC, MD, MBA
Vice Chair for Clinical Pathology and Quality, Department of Pathology, Director of Clinical Laboratories, Brigham and Women's Hospital, Dana-Farber Cancer Institute, Associate Professor of Pathology, Harvard Medical School, Boston, Massachusetts, USA

EDITOR

GEZA S. BODOR, MD
Professor, Department of Pathology, Director, Toxicology and TDM, University of Colorado Anschutz Medical Campus, Aurora, Colorado, USA

AUTHORS

GEZA S. BODOR, MD
Professor, Department of Pathology, Director, Toxicology and TDM, University of Colorado Anschutz Medical Campus, Aurora, Colorado, USA

CORY BYSTROM, PhD
Research and Development, Cleveland HeartLab, Cleveland, Ohio, USA

ANDREW E. CLARK, PhD
University of Arizona, Tucson, Arizona, USA

CHRISTA M. COBBAERT, PhD
Department of Clinical Chemistry and Laboratory Medicine, Leiden University Medical Center (LUMC), Leiden, The Netherlands

ROBERT L. FITZGERALD, PhD, DABCC/T
Professor, Department of Pathology, Director, Toxicology/Mass Spectrometry Laboratory, University of California, San Diego, University of California, San Diego Health System, Center for Advanced Laboratory Medicine, San Diego, California, USA

UTTAM GARG, PhD
Director, Division of Laboratory Medicine, Professor, Department of Pathology and Laboratory Medicine, Children's Mercy Hospital, University of Missouri Health School of Medicine, Kansas City, Missouri, USA

MARK S. LOWENTHAL, PhD
Material Measurement Laboratory, Biomolecular Measurement Division, National Institute of Standards and Technology (NIST), Gaithersburg, Maryland, USA

KARA L. LYNCH, PhD
Associate Professor, Department of Laboratory Medicine, Clinical Laboratory,
Zuckerberg San Francisco General Hospital, University of California, San Francisco,
San Francisco, California, USA

BRIAN A. RAPPOLD, PhD
Laboratory Corporation of America, Durham, North Carolina, USA

ALAN L. ROCKWOOD, PhD, DABCC
Rockwood Scientific Consulting, Salt Lake City, Utah, USA

JUDITH A. STONE, MT(ASCP), PhD, DABCC
Senior Technical Specialist, Toxicology/Mass Spectrometry Laboratory, University
of California, San Diego Health System, Center for Advanced Laboratory Medicine,
San Diego, California, USA

NICOLE V. TOLAN, PhD, DABCC
Assistant Adjunct Professor, Pathology and Laboratory Medicine, Tufts University School
of Medicine, Boston, Massachusetts, USA; SCIEX Diagnostics, Director, Scientific and
Medical Affairs, Framingham, Massachusetts, USA

YURI E.M. VAN DER BURGT, PhD
Department of Clinical Chemistry and Laboratory Medicine, Center for Proteomics and
Metabolomics, Leiden University Medical Center (LUMC), Leiden, The Netherlands

DONNA M. WOLK, MHA, PhD, D(ABMM)
System Director, Clinical Microbiology, Diagnostic Medicine Institute, Department of
Laboratory Medicine, Geisinger Health, Danville, Pennsylvania, USA; Wilkes University,
Wilkes-Barre, Pennsylvania, USA

Contents

Vitamin D has been associated with many health conditions. Because of widespread deficiency in the general population, laboratory testing of vitamin D has increased exponentially in recent years. Currently, 25-hydroxyvitamin D (25[OH]D) is considered the best marker of vitamin D status. Automated immunoassays and tandem mass spectrometry are the most widely used assays for the measurement of 25(OH)D. Because a medical decision of vitamin D deficiency and treatment are made based on specific levels, it is important that different 25(OH)D assays are harmonized. Despite standardization efforts, significant differences remain among various methods and laboratories for the measurement of 25(OH)D.

For appropriate pain medication monitoring, the analytical method must be sensitive enough to detect the prescribed medication and metabolites at a sufficiently low concentration to recognize compliance, even with a low-dose prescription. The method must also provide excellent selectivity to identify simultaneously present drugs even with similar chemical structures. The analytical method should uncover common illicit drugs/nonprescribed medications. Traditional immunoassays cannot satisfy these criteria, but liquid chromatography tandem mass spectrometry can. It requires expensive instrumentation, careful test design, and extensive validation and produces a large amount of data that must be interpreted according to the clinical context.

Matrix-assisted laser desorption time of flight mass spectrometry (MALDI-TOF MS), adapted for use in clinical microbiology laboratories, challenges current standards of microbial detection and identification. This article summarizes the capabilities of MALDI-TOF MS in diagnostic clinical microbiology laboratories and describes the underpinnings of the technology, highlighting topics such as sample preparation, spectral analysis, and accuracy. The use of MALDI-TOF MS in the clinical microbiology laboratory is growing, and, when properly deployed, can accelerate diagnosis and improve patient care.

In clinical testing of protein markers, structure variants of the measurand are often not taken into account. This heterogeneous character of protein measurands in immunoassays often renders test standardization impossible. Consequently, test results from different methods can lead to underdiagnosis or overdiagnosis and, thus, undertreatment or overtreatment of patients. The systematic structural analysis of protein isoforms has been coined proteoform profiling and is performed through mass spectrometry–based proteomics strategies. Knowledge on proteoforms allows refining existing unimarker tests and moreover has great potential to contribute to the urgent need for new tests to predict prognosis and severity of diseases.

Harmonization of diagnostic test results is fundamental to the effective use of laboratory testing in the diagnosis, treatment, and monitoring of disease. Formal approaches to harmonization and standardization provide a rigorous and high-quality roadmap to this end, although the formal harmonization process can be long and complex. In the meantime, more informal approaches to harmonization can provide a useful pathway to improved harmonization in the short term. Factors relevant to harmonization are discussed with particular attention to protein assays using LC-MS/MS. Published formal and informal harmonization projects are provided as examples, including lessons drawn from these projects.

For mass spectrometry (MS) testing in the clinical laboratory, postimplementation monitoring for quality is just as important as method development and validation but often receives less attention. Quality-assurance monitoring for liquid chromatography–tandem MS (LC-MS/MS) testing should be proactive rather than reactive and should monitor the entire testing process. An LC-MS/MS quality-assurance plan should cover overall batch review parameters, individual peak review parameters, system and reagent changes, and assessment of long-term accuracy. This article discusses Clinical Laboratory Improvement Amendments' regulations as they apply to LC-MS/MS–based testing and reviews available guidelines for LC-MS/MS quality assurance and postimplementation monitoring.

This article describes the need for, stratifies the complexity of, and proposes detailed lists of training competencies for diagnostic laboratory personnel using quantitative liquid chromatography–tandem mass spectrometry (LC-MS/MS) for patient care. Although quantitative LC-MS/MS is evolving toward greater automation with less need for technical expertise, gaps remain in resources for training and assessment.

Special Considerations for Liquid Chromatography–Tandem Mass Spectrometry Method Development

Brian A. Rappold

Method development for diagnostic liquid chromatography–tandem mass spectrometry (LC-MS/MS) assays are not broadly discussed in publications. Certain aspects of the development process are thus learned via experience. This article touches on a number of aspects that should be contemplated during method development for LC-MS/MS tests beyond sample preparation, chromatographic separation, and mass spectrometric detection. Utilization of factors intrinsic to LC-MS/MS, such as isotopically labeled internal standards and appraisal of transition ratios, engenders confidence in assay development and accelerates movement toward validation and testing.

Development of a 25-Hydroxyvitamin D Liquid Chromatography–Tandem Mass Spectrometry Assay, Cleared by the Food and Drug Administration, via the De Novo Pathway

Nicole V. Tolan

Despite great improvement in vitamin D assay standardization, inaccurate recoveries of $25(OH)D_2$ remain for immunoassays, and many laboratory-developed LC-MS/MS methods do not separate out the 3-epimer interferents. Through the process of obtaining Food and Drug Administration (FDA) clearance, we learned that communication is key. Mass spectrometry–based assays raise different questions of safety and efficacy than the predicate immunoassays, with fewer risks due to increased accuracy. This process required improving our quality management system to support the development and registration of an in vitro diagnostic device. There are similar examples for a number of analytes, requiring expeditious entry of FDA-cleared LC-MS/MS methods into clinical laboratories.

CLINICS IN LABORATORY MEDICINE

SERIES OF RELATED INTEREST

Surgical Pathology Clinics
Available at: http://www.surgpath.theclinics.com

THE CLINICS ARE NOW AVAILABLE ONLINE!
Access your subscription at:
www.theclinics.com

Preface

It's Mass Spectrometry's Turn to Change Clinical Practice

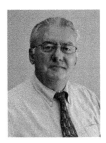

Geza S. Bodor, MD
Editor

Norbert Elias in his essay, *Scientific Establishments*, used the metaphor of a spiral staircase to illustrate the advancement of human knowledge. Medical science follows this mode of advancement. Existing knowledge and technology are applied to unanswered questions, extending our pool of information and refining our understanding, but eventually, the capabilities of existing technology reach their limits, and while illuminating previously dark areas of the discipline, they also leave behind more unanswered questions requiring newer, more sophisticated technology to probe these territories. Thus, a new cycle begins.

The history of laboratory medicine provides an excellent demonstration of this spiral advancement process. "Sensory diagnostics" (taste, smell, and color) was superseded by simple chemical reactions followed by the measurement of enzyme activity and eventually immunoassays. Approximately two decades ago, we started applying molecular genetic methods on a wide scale that is now expanded into whole-genome and single-cell nucleic acid analyses, and we are examining the options to use gene editing tools for diagnosis. The most recent technical development in laboratory medicine is employing a relatively old analytical method, mass spectrometry (MS), in combination with other analytical methods, to make new inquiries about biochemical and pathologic processes in the human body. The new technology is drastically changing the practice of laboratory diagnostics. MS has started the new revolution in the literal and figurative sense of the word.

MS uses basic physical principles such as molecular mass, charge, and time to ascertain characteristics of molecules in human samples to derive diagnostic conclusions. The high analytical sensitivity of this method allows detection of previously unseen components, and its unparalleled resolution allows us to dissect seemingly uniform mixtures of molecules. These two characteristics of the technology permit simultaneous measurement of multiple analytes that may differ only by a single proton.

Clin Lab Med 38 (2018) ix–xi
https://doi.org/10.1016/j.cll.2018.06.001
0272-2712/18/© 2018 Published by Elsevier Inc.

labmed.theclinics.com

Finally, MS can do all these "miracles" without requiring alteration, for instance, derivatization, of the molecule under examination. Because modification or prior amplification of very low concentration constituents is not needed, the chance for misidentification of detected chemicals or missing the presence of important substances is minimized.

MS can also be combined with other advanced analytical techniques, such as gas or liquid chromatography (LC), to enhance resolution and selectivity. This linked technology, in the form of gas chromatography MS, was among the earliest applications of mass spectrometers in the clinical toxicology laboratory. Atmospheric pressure ionization was needed to allow the use of the liquid chromatograph for separation of sample mixtures before MS analysis, forming the LC-MS. Because atmospheric pressure ionization produces soft ionization, multiple mass spectrometers in tandem (tandem MS or MS/MS) had to be used to break up the ions in the machine for analysis of the fragments, facilitating positive analyte identification. However, prior chromatographic separation of molecules is not essential, and several other sample introduction practices are now utilized, including direct infusion, gas phase sample introduction, paper spray, or various desorption methods that are combined with ionization, such as in matrix-assisted laser desorption ionization, to mention a few. The tandem MS is only one of the various mass spectrometers now in use by clinical laboratories. Ion traps can be included in the tandem MS, and physical properties of ions can be exploited for identification of molecules, as in accurate mass MS, represented by the time-of-flight (TOF) or orbitrap instruments. These techniques are complementary and may have specific uses in special circumstances. With proper selection of the analytical techniques, it is now possible to measure analytes of several thousands of Daltons mass range at picomole (10^{-12}) to femtomole (10^{-15}) concentrations.

Many articles in this issue of the *Clinics in Laboratory Medicine* describe current uses of mass spectrometers in the clinical laboratory. The selection of these examples is arbitrary but with the goal to show a cross-section of clinical applications and necessities. A comprehensive representation of all types of clinical applications is impossible within the scope of this publication. Small molecule testing is the most prevalent MS function in clinical MS, and several articles are included here on this topic. Other articles investigate the current state of proteomic analysis by LC-MSMS and discuss the use of TOF MS in the microbiology lab. The rapid development of mass spectrometric methods by independent laboratories without the help of certified analytical standards introduces new problems: the potential lack of agreement between results of different origins. Transferability of results obtained from different laboratories is imperative for continuity of patient care; therefore, MS result standardization must be undertaken, either by between-laboratory cooperation, by the development and application of international standards, or by test approval by regulatory agencies such as the Food and Drug Administration. Several reports in this issue explore the current status of assay standardization via one of these processes, while also pointing out necessary actions to expedite the standardization procedures to keep pace with the rapid spread of MS methods into clinical diagnosis.

The authors of the articles are accomplished researchers, and they are also directors of clinical MS laboratories. They have many years of experience developing and validating new diagnostic assays, and their practical experience is reflected in the articles, whether written on testing specific analytes, describing how to develop robust analytical methods, providing guidance toward accreditation of an MS laboratory, or setting goals for the training of MS laboratory personnel. In addition to MS laboratory operation specifics, the readers will find extensive references with the articles aiding medical and technical directors to start and maintain high-quality MS laboratories, but policy-makers at regulatory agencies and industry representatives can also find valuable information in this issue of the *Clinics in Laboratory Medicine*. The articles also guide pathology residency and fellowship program directors and other educators on what to include in the necessary curriculum to properly train future specialists for clinical MS.

This issue of the *Clinics in Laboratory Medicine* will show how far the MS revolution advanced in a relatively short period of time and will also provide guidance on what needs to be accomplished to fully integrate MS into the clinical laboratory diagnostic process. Promising recent results of novel applications of MS are not covered because of publication limits and because many of these results are at the level of proof of concept experiments at this time. It is hoped that a future issue of the *Clinics in Laboratory Medicine* will present those findings as they gain acceptance into clinical practice after additional testing and evaluation.

Geza S. Bodor, MD
Department of Pathology
University of Colorado
Anschutz Medical Campus
Leprino Building, Room 229
Mail Stop A022
12401 East 17th Avenue
Aurora, CO 80045, USA

E-mail address:
geza.bodor@ucdenver.edu

25-Hydroxyvitamin D Testing

Immunoassays Versus Tandem Mass Spectrometry

Uttam Garg, PhD

KEYWORDS

- Vitamin D • 25-Hydroxyvitamin D • HPLC-tandem mass spectrometry
- HPLC-MS/MS • Vitamin D binding-protein • Immunoassay • Protein-binding assay
- 3-Epi-25-hydroxyvitamin D

KEY POINTS

- In addition to playing a vital role in bone health, vitamin D has been associated with many other health conditions, such as diabetes, cardiovascular diseases, cancer, multiple sclerosis, and immune system functions.
- Several epidemiologic studies have shown that the prevalence of vitamin D deficiency is widespread in the general population.
- Although, 1,25-dihydroxyvitamin D is the active form of vitamin D, 25-hydroxyvitamin D is the best marker of vitamin D status.
- Immunoassays and HPLC-MS/MS are the most widely used techniques for the assay of 25-hydroxyvitamin D.
- Despite standardization efforts, significant differences remain among different methods for the measurement of 25-hydroxyvitamin D.

INTRODUCTION

Two major forms of vitamin D are cholecalciferol (vitamin D_3) and ergocalciferol (vitamin D_2). Vitamin D_3 is synthesized in the skin from the precursor 7-dehydrocholesterol by cutaneous exposure to ultraviolet (UV) B radiation of wavelength 295 to 300 nm. Vitamin D_3 is also derived from oil-rich fish, such as salmon, mackerel, and herring. Vitamin D_2 is synthesized from UV irradiation of the yeast sterol ergosterol and is also found naturally in sun-exposed mushrooms. Both vitamin D_3 and vitamin D_2 are used in food fortification and vitamin D supplements. Vitamin D, synthesized

Disclosure: The author has nothing to disclose.
Department of Pathology and Laboratory Medicine, Children's Mercy Hospital, University of Missouri School of Medicine, 2401 Gillham Road, Kansas City, MO 64108, USA
E-mail address: ugarg@cmh.edu

Clin Lab Med 38 (2018) 439–453
https://doi.org/10.1016/j.cll.2018.05.007
0272-2712/18/© 2018 Elsevier Inc. All rights reserved.

labmed.theclinics.com

in the skin or consumed through diet, is metabolized in the liver to 25-hydroxyvitamin D (25[OH]D) by vitamin D-25-hydroxylase. In the kidneys, 25(OH)D is converted to 1,25-dihydroxyvitamin D (1,25[OH]2D), an active form of vitamin D, by 25(OH)D-1-α-hydroxylase. Vitamin D and its metabolites are transported to various tissues primarily by a vitamin D binding-protein (VDBP), although albumin and lipoproteins are also important transporters. 1,25(OH)2D binds to its receptors, which are present in most tissues and cells in the body.

In addition to playing a vital role in bone health, vitamin D has been associated with other health conditions, such as diabetes, cardiovascular diseases, cancer, multiple sclerosis, and immune system functions.[1,2] Nutritional deficiency and lack of sun exposure are the major causes of vitamin D deficiency. Certain pathophysiologic conditions, such as intestinal malabsorption, renal disease, and liver failure, also cause vitamin D deficiency. In recent years, several epidemiologic studies have shown that the prevalence of vitamin D deficiency is widespread in the general population. This has led to a massive rise in laboratory testing for the assessment of vitamin D deficiency. Although 1,25-dihydroxyvitamin D is the active form of vitamin D, 25(OH)D is the principal circulating form of vitamin D and is currently considered the best marker of vitamin D status. Measurement of 1,25(OH)2D is only recommended in certain conditions, such as acquired and inherited disorders of vitamin D and phosphate metabolism.

Various methods including immunoassays, competitive protein-binding assays (CPBA), high-performance liquid chromatography (HPLC)-UV, and HPLC-tandem mass spectrometry (HPLC-MS/MS) are used for the measurement of 25(OH)D. Because of automation, low start-up costs, and smaller sample volume, immunoassays are the most widely used methods for the assay of 25(OH)D. HPLC-MS/MS is considered the gold standard for the measurement of 25(OH)D. Advantages of HPLC-MS/MS include increased specificity and the ability to differentiate 25(OH)D3 and 25(OH)D2.

25-HYDROXYVITAMIN D REFERENCE INTERVALS

Currently, 25(OH)D is considered the best indicator of the vitamin D status because contrarily to 1,25(OH)2D, its level is not dependent on parathyroid harmone (PTH) concentration and it shows low intraindividual variability because of its longer half-life of approximately 3 weeks. Unlike other vitamins, population-based vitamin D reference ranges cannot be established. This is because several factors including season of the year, gender, ethnicity, sunlight exposure, diet, age, gender, body mass index, and skin pigmentation affect vitamin D concentrations. 25(OH)D reference ranges based on health and disease are, therefore, more appropriate than the traditional central 95% values from healthy individuals.

Regarding optimal 25(OH)D concentrations, certain agreements and disagreements remain among vitamin D experts. Most experts agree that 25(OH)D concentrations lower than 20 ng/mL are associated with poor bone health. There is no consensus, however, on the optimal concentrations of 25(OH)D.[3–6] Also, there is no unanimity on the toxic concentrations of 25(OH)D; levels up to 80 ng/mL are generally considered safe. The Institute of Medicine and Endocrine Society recommended reference ranges are provided in **Table 1**.[4,7] These differences in 25(OH)D are large enough to classify a significant number of individuals at risk of vitamin D deficiency or not. Following these guidelines, an international meeting of vitamin D experts held in Warsaw, Poland in 2012 concluded that target concentration for 25(OH)D should be 30 to 50 ng/mL.[8] Recent Japanese guidelines define 25(OH)D levels of less than 20 ng/mL as deficient, 20 to 30 ng/mL as insufficient, and 30 to 60 ng/mL as sufficient.[9]

Table 1
Institute of Medicine and Endocrine Society Guidelines for interpreting the concentration of serum total 25(OH)D

Category	Institute of Medicine, General Population, ng/mL	Endocrine Society Population at Risk, ng/mL
Deficiency	<12	<20
Insufficiency	12–20	20–29
Sufficiency	20–30	30–100
No added benefit	30–50	—
Possible harm	>50	>100

Note: to convert ng/mL to nmol/L multiply ng/mL value by 2.5.
Data from Holick MF, Binkley NC, Bischoff-Ferrari HA, et al. Evaluation, treatment, and prevention of vitamin D deficiency: an Endocrine Society clinical practice guideline. J Clin Endocrinol Metab 2011;96:1911–30; and Ross AC. The 2011 report on dietary reference intakes for calcium and vitamin D. Public Health Nutr 2011;14:938–9.

HARMONIZATION OF 25-HYDROXYVITAMIN D ASSAYS

Because medical decisions regarding vitamin D deficiency are based on the specific values of 25(OH)D, it is important that different methods for the measurement of 25(OH)D are comparable and harmonized. Various studies have shown that accurate measurement of 25(OH)D is challenging and there are clinically significant differences among various 25(OH)D assays. Many factors including the inconsistent release of 25(OH)D from VDBP and its similarity with many other endogenous compounds have contributed to these analytical challenges. 25(OH)D is a highly lipophilic molecule and is strongly associated with VDBP. Releasing and extracting 25(OH)D from VDBP can lead to coextraction of endogenous lipids that may affect ligand binding and chromatographic methods. Another challenge in the accurate measurement of 25(OH)D is the presence of isobaric compounds or other vitamin D metabolites that may cross-react with antibodies or may not be separated chromatographically.

In response to poor performance and large variability among 25(OH)D assays, several quality assessment programs were initiated. One such large program, the Vitamin D External Quality Assessment Scheme (DEQAS), was established in 1989 to monitor the performance of 25(OH)D assays. Monitoring of other vitamin D metabolites 1,25- dihydroxyvitamin D, 24,25-dihydroxyvitamin D, and 3-epi-25(OH)D, was introduced in later years.[10,11] In 2010, the Vitamin D Standardization Program (VDSP) was initiated by the National Institutes of Health Office of Dietary Supplements. College of American Pathologists (CAP) also offers an accuracy-based external proficiency survey for the assessment of 25(OH)D. In addition, the Centers for Disease Control and Prevention (CDC) provides a Vitamin D Standardization-Certification Program to certify laboratories based on accurate measurements of 25(OH)D. The major objective of these programs is to standardize the laboratory measurements (commercial, clinical, and research) of 25(OH)D to reference measurement procedures (RMPs) developed by the National Institute for Standards and Technology (NIST), Ghent University, and the CDC. These programs have resulted in significant improvement in the performance of 25(OH)D assays resulting in increased accuracy and a reduction in variability among different laboratories and assays. This is evident from the DEQAS survey data collected over the years. In 1989, interlaboratory CVs ranged from 29.3% to 53.7% and decreased to 10.3% to 15.3% in 2017.[10]

Production and availability of reference materials has been the key to standardization and improving the accuracy and precision of 25(OH)D assays. NIST, in collaboration with National Institutes of Health Office of Dietary Supplements, produced several standard reference materials (SRMs). Commercial availability of these SRMs facilitated validation and the harmonization of various 25(OH)D assays. SRM 972a contains four human-serum-based solutions containing different concentrations (20–80 nmol/L) of 25(OH)D3, 25(OH)D2, 3-epi-25(OH)D3, and 24,25(OH)2D3. More recently, human-serum-based solution, SRM 2973, with a total 25(OH)D concentration near 100 nmol/L was released to complement SRM 972a. SRM 2973 also contains 25(OH)D3, 25(OH)D2, 3-epi-25(OH)D3, and 24,25(OH)2D3. In addition to SRM 972a and SRM 2973, which are human-serum-based solutions, ethanol-based SRM 2972a is also commercially available. SRM 2972a is intended primarily for use in the calibration of instruments and techniques used for the determination of vitamin D metabolites.

Originally, the quality assessment programs compared the participants' results with peer-group means or all-laboratory trimmed mean (ALTM). In DEQAS, ALTM was a good surrogate for the true 25(OH)D value; ALTM values compared well with the 25(OH)D gas chromatography–mass spectrometry method.[10,11] Now all DEQAS and CAP external quality control samples are assigned 25(OH)D values using RMPs. Participants' results are compared with the assigned values rather than peer method-based or ALTM values. To achieve an acceptable annual performance on DEQAS, 75% of participants' results must be within 25% of the true values for 25(OH)D3 + 25(OH)D2, as determined by the NIST RMP. In CAP ABVD surveys, acceptable performance requires participant values within 25% or 5 ng/mL, whichever is greater, of the CDC reference value.

25-HYDROXYVITAMIN D ASSAYS

There are two major categories of 25(OH)D assays: nonchromatographic methods involving 25(OH)D binding protein or antibody, and chromatographic methods.[12] Before 1990, only a limited number of laboratories performed 25(OH)D assays. These laboratories used in-house CPBA or HPLC with UV detection. CPBA with and without chromatographic separation of 25(OH)D were developed. These assays were laborious and many suffered from inaccuracy, poor sensitivity, imprecision, and unequal cross-reactivity with 25(OH)D2 and 25(OH)D3. Because of these limitations, earlier CPBAs were discontinued and were predominantly replaced by radioimmunoassays (RIAs). RIAs used polyclonal antibodies raised against 25(OH)D. Earlier, RIAs also suffered from poor extraction, imprecision, inaccuracies, and unequal cross-reactivity of antibodies with 25(OH)D2 and 25(OH)D3. In 1993, Hollis and colleagues[13] developed an RIA based on serum raised against the 23,24,25,26,27-pentanor-C-(22)-carboxylic acid vitamin D-BSA conjugate. The assay claimed approximately 100% cross-reactivity with 25(OH)D2 and 25(OH)D3. This assay led to the development of the first commercial RIA for the measurement of 25(OH)D marketed by DiaSorin (Stillwater, MN). It was a two-step method involving 25(OH)D extraction and a competitive immunoassay involving iodinated 25(OH)D tracer. DiaSorin RIA was used in several clinical studies and public health surveys and to establish 25(OH)D reference ranges. Immuno Diagnostics Systems (United Kingdom) also developed a commercial RIA.

With increased test volume, most clinical laboratories abandoned manual CPBA and RIA in favor of commercial automated CPBA and nonradioactive immunoassays. To achieve accuracy and precision, these assays have to maintain a delicate balance between releasing 25(OH)D from VDBP and its binding to antibodies or specific proteins. Over the years, a large number of CPBA or immunoassays have been commercially developed. DEQAS, which is the world's largest external quality assessment program with more than 1000 participants from 56 countries, provides a good glance on the development of various 25(OH)D methods. **Table 2** provides the timeline on the introduction of various 25(OH)D assays.[10,11] Currently, DEQAS receives data from greater than 30 different 25(OH)D methods. In July 2017, commonly used methods (N >30) by DEQAS participants were DiaSorin Liaison Total (n = 214), Roche Total (n = 165), Siemens ADVIA Centaur (n = 165), HPLC-MS/MS (n = 159), Abbott Architect New Kit (n = 71), IDS-iSYS (n = 63), and Beckman Unicel Dxi (n = 32). A major change in the method usage over the last 10 years is a significant increase in HPLC-MS/MS and automated CPBA or immunoassays, and a decrease in manual methods.

A large number of participants and methods in DEQAS make the data analysis robust. In addition to assessing the accuracy of 25(OH)D methods, large data provides opportunity to study the other aspects, such as linearity, specificity, and the effect of anticoagulants. DEQAS data revealed that 25(OH)D results by different methods had been erratic but showed significant improvement in the accuracy and precision. In April 2017, five out of six fully automated assays, 93.3% HPLC and 91.3% HPLC-MS/MS, had a bias within the VDSP limits.

HPLC-UV detection has remained in use for many decades but has largely been replaced by HPLC-MS/MS. Currently, the most commonly used methods for the measurement of 25(OH)D are automated immunoassays and HPLC-MS/MS. It is estimated that approximately 70% of 25(OH)D testing is performed using automated methods and approximately 15% by HPLC-MS/MS techniques. Although

Table 2
Timeline for 25(OH)D methods as they first appeared in DEQAS

Date	Method
Oct 1989	CPB
April 1991	HPLC (22)
April 1993	IncStar RIA
July 1999	DiaSorin RIA (1)
	IDS RIA (5)
July 2001	Nichols Advantage
Oct 2002	IDS EIA (OCTEIA) (13)
April 2004	DiaSorin Liaison
Oct 2005	LC-MS/MS (160)
April 2007	DiaSorin Liaison Total (226)
Oct 2007	Roche 25(OH)D
Jan 2009	IDS iSYS (80)
Jan 2011	Abbott Architect (83)
April 2011	Siemens ADVIA Centaur (68)
	Roche Total 25(OH)D (170)
Jan 2014	Beckman Unicel Dxi Total 25(OH)D (33)

Number of results submitted in January 2017 are in parenthesis.
Data from Carter GD, Berry J, Durazo-Arvizu R, et al. Hydroxyvitamin D assays: an historical perspective from DEQAS. J Steroid Biochem Mol Biol 2018;177:30–5; and Carter GD, Jones JC, Shannon J, et al. 25-Hydroxyvitamin D assays: potential interference from other circulating vitamin D metabolites. J Steroid Biochem Mol Biol 2016;164:134–8.

immunoassays are widely used in routine practice, HPLC-MS/MS is considered the gold standard method for the measurement of 25(OH)D. The technology is used by NIST, CDC, and VDSP to assign values to vitamin D metabolites. Advantages and limitations of automated and HPLC-MS/MS methods are discussed in **Table 3**.

AUTOMATED IMMUNOASSAYS AND PROTEIN-BINDING ASSAYS FOR 25-HYDROXYVITAMIN D

Several Food and Drug Administration (FDA) approved automated immunoassays and protein-binding assays are available for the determination of 25(OH)D. These assays are available on major chemistry platforms and provide rapid turnaround time. Unlike chromatographic methods, automated assays are simple to use, often require low sample volume, and do not need a large initial capital cost and specialized expertise. Most of these assays are competitive immunoassays or protein-binding assays based on chemiluminescent technology. A common step in these assays is the pretreatment of patient samples with denaturing agents to release 25(OH)D from VDBP. This is followed by the addition of immobilized anti-25(OH)D-antibody or vitamin D protein-binding. Subsequently, 25(OH)D with a tag that binds to the unbound sites is added to the mixture. A signal produced by the tag is inversely proportional to the 25(OH)D concentration in the patient sample. Principles of commonly used automated assays are discussed next.

DiaSorin Liaison 25(OH)D is a direct competitive chemiluminescent immunoassay. In the first step, 25(OH)D released from VDBP binds to the specific antibody on the solid phase. In the next step, vitamin D linked to an isoluminol derivative is added. Subsequently, the unbound material is washed away, and starter reagents are added to initiate chemiluminescent reaction. The chemiluminescent signal is inversely proportional to the concentration of 25(OH)D present in the samples.

The Roche 25(OH)D assay is a competitive chemiluminescent VDBP assay. 25(OH)D released from the sample is incubated with ruthenium-labelled VDBP. This is followed by the addition of streptavidin-coated microparticles and 25(OH)D labeled with biotin, which binds to unoccupied sites on ruthenium-labelled VDBP. A complex consisting of ruthenylated VDBP and the biotinylated 25(OH)D is formed and becomes bound to the solid phase via interaction of biotin and streptavidin. Microparticles are magnetically captured onto the surface of the electrode and unbound material is

Table 3
Advantages and disadvantages of immunoassays and HPLC-MS/MS

	Advantages	Disadvantages
Immunoassays	• Smaller sample volume • High-throughput • Automation • High sensitivity • Low start-up cost • Technically simple	• Lower specificity • Cross-reactivity with vitamin D metabolites • Cannot distinguish vitamin D_2 and D_3 • Extraction of 25(OH)D may be challenging
HPLC-MS/MS	• High specificity • Can distinguish 25(OH)D2 and 25(OH)D3 • Separation of vitamin D metabolites • Reference method	• Most methods do not separate epimers • Expensive start-up cost • Technically more demanding, need expertise • Automation challenging

removed. The application of a voltage to the electrode induces chemiluminescent emission, which is inversely proportional to the 25(OH)D concentration in the sample.

The Siemens ADVIA Centaur 25(OH)D assay is a competitive immunoassay that uses an antifluorescein monoclonal mouse antibody covalently bound to paramagnetic particles, an anti-25(OH)D monoclonal mouse antibody labeled with acridinium ester, and a vitamin D analogue labeled with fluorescein. An inverse relationship exists between the amount of 25(OH)D present in the patient sample and the amount of relative light units detected by the system.

The ARCHITECT 25(OH)D assay is a competitive chemiluminescent microparticle immunoassay. In the first step, a sample is incubated with 25(OH)D releasing agent and paramagnetic anti-vitamin-D-coated microparticles. 25(OH)D present in the sample binds to anti–vitamin D antibodies coated microparticles. This is followed by the addition of acridinium-labeled 25(OH)D, which binds to unoccupied sites. After washing the unbound material, pretrigger and trigger solutions are added and chemiluminescence is measured. The amount of vitamin D in the sample is inversely proportional to the chemiluminescence signal.

The IDS-iSYS 25(OH)D assay is a competitive chemiluminescent immunoassay. The patient sample is subjected to a pretreatment step to denature the VDBP and release 25(OH)D. The treated samples are then neutralized in assay buffer and the anti-25(OH)D antibody, labeled with biotin, is added to the mixture. After incubation, acridinium-labeled 25(OH)D is added. Subsequently, magnetic particles linked to streptavidin are added. In the final step, magnetic particles are separated and unbound analyte washed. Trigger reagents are added to generate light from acridinium label. The light generated is inversely proportional to the concentration of 25(OH)D in the sample.

The Beckman Coulter 25(OH)D assay is a two-step competitive binding immunoenzymatic assay. In the first step, the sample is incubated with 25(OH)D releasing agent and paramagnetic particles coated with sheep monoclonal anti-25(OH)D antibody. Released 25(OH)D binds to the immobilized monoclonal anti-25(OH)D antibody. Subsequently, a 25(OH)D analogue-alkaline phosphatase conjugate is added, which competes for binding to the immobilized monoclonal anti-25(OH)D antibody. Unbound material is washed away and chemiluminescent substrate is added. The chemiluminescent light production is inversely proportional to the concentration of 25(OH)D in the sample.

The VITROS 25(OH)D assay is a competitive chemiluminescent immunoassay. 25(OH)D in the sample is released using a low pH denaturant. Subsequently, 25(OH)D in the sample and horseradish peroxidase–labeled 25(OH)D compete for monoclonal anti-25(OH)D bound to the wells. Unbound materials are removed by washing. The bound horseradish peroxidase conjugate is measured by a luminescent reaction. The amount of horseradish peroxidase conjugate bound is indirectly proportional to the concentration of 25(OH)D.

Characteristics of several commercially available automated immunoassays are shown in **Table 4**. Of note, many of these assays show significant cross-reactivity with 24,25(OH)2D3 and C-3 epi-25(OH)D3.

CHROMATOGRAPHIC ASSAYS FOR 25-HYDROXYVITAMIN D

Chromatographic methods have been widely used for the assay of 25(OH)D and other metabolites of vitamin D. These methods offer several advantages, the most obvious being the separation and simultaneous measurement of several clinically relevant vitamin D metabolites, such as 25(OH)D3, 25(OH)D2, 1,25(OH)2D3, 1,25(OH)2D2, 24,25(OH)2D3, 24,25(OH)2D2, and 3-epi-25(OH)D. HPLC with UV detection, first

Table 4
Characteristics of various commercial immunoassays

Commercial Assay	Test Principle	Linear Range, ng/mL	Imprecision, Various Levels, %	Cross-Reactivity, %				
				25(OH)D3	25(OH)D2	24,25(OH)2D3	24,25(OH)2D2	C3-epimer of 25(OH)D
DiaSorin liaison total	Competitive chemiluminescent immunoassay	4–151	6–13	100	100	No mention	No mention	1
Roche elecsys	Competitive chemiluminescent protein-binding assay	5–60	2–13	100	92	149	No mention	91
Siemens ADVIA centaur	Competitive chemiluminescent immunoassay	4–150	4–12	101	105	No mention	No mention	1
Abbott architect new kit	Competitive chemiluminescent immunoassay	3–156	2–7	100	81	102–189	71–149	1
IDS-iSYS	Competitive chemiluminescent immunoassay	7–125	6–12	97	120	124	No mention	1
Beckman unicel Dxi	Competitive chemiluminescent immunoassay	7–120	7–9	100	86–103	3–16	No mention	100
Vitros ECi/ECiQ	Competitive chemiluminescent immunoassay	13–126	5–16	99	105	35	No mention	37

described in 1978, was an earlier chromatographic method for the assay of vitamin D metabolites. HPLC coulometric electrochemical detection method based on the oxidation potential of the conjugated-diene structure of vitamin D metabolites has also been described. Although the electrochemical detection method is comparable with HPLC-UV, it has not gained popularity because of its high maintenance. In recent years, there has been a major shift toward the use of HPLC-MS/MS. HPLC-MS/MS has several advantages over immunoassays and HPLC-UV. In addition to chromatographic separation, HPLC-MS/MS provides increased selectivity through the analysis of specific mass-to-charge ratios (m/z) of different compounds. In mass spectrometry, accuracy and precision are further improved by the use of stable isotope-labelled internal standards.

Several HPLC-UV and HPLC-MS/MS methods for the assay of 25(OH)D and other clinically relevant metabolites of vitamin D have been described. Earlier HPLC-UV methods used silica columns, which have been primarily replaced by more stable and robust reverse phase C18 columns. A typical HPLC-UV method for the assay of 25(OH)D3 and 25(OH)D2 has been described by Lensmeyer and colleagues.[14] The method involved extraction of 25(OH)D using Strata-X (surface-modified styrene-divinylbenzene resin) extraction cartridges (Phenomenex) and acetonitrile/water. The extracts are dried at 35°C with a stream of nitrogen, reconstituted in ethyl acetate/acetonitrile, and injected in HPLC-UV system. The HPLC-UV system consisted of a guard column, an analytical column (5-μm Stable BondTM Cyanopropyl, Agilent Technologies), and UV detector set at 275 nm. Columns temperature was 50°C, and the mobile phase was methanol/water (67:33 vol/vol). The method was linear from 5 to 200 ng/mL with recoveries from 95% to 102%. Between-run CVs were 2.6% to 4.9% for 25(OH)D3 and 3.2% to 13% for 25(OH)D2. The method was compared with HPLC-MS/MS, a CPBA on the Nichols Advantage platform and an RIA from DiaSorin.

HPLC-MS/MS methods for the measurement of vitamin D metabolites include fast atom bombardment, electrospray ionization, and atmospheric pressure chemical ionization.[15–23] Because vitamin D metabolites are nonpolar, atmospheric pressure chemical ionization may provide better results compared with electrospray ionization. A typical HPLC-MS/MS method for the measurement of vitamin D metabolites consists of the addition of stable isotope-labelled internal standards, protein denaturation to release vitamin D from VDBP, liquid-liquid or solid phase extraction, drying of extracts, and reconstitution of extracts for injection in HPLC-MS/MS. Methods involving direct protein precipitation and the injection of supernatants into HPLC-MS/MS have also been described. These direct methods may show higher ion-suppression, but their accuracy and precision are generally not effected when stable isotope internal standards are used. A direct protein precipitation method used in our laboratory is briefly described.[16] In this method, acetonitrile containing internal standard 25(OH)D3-d6 (26, 26, 26, 27, 27, 27-d6) is added to the sample. The mixture is vortexed and left at room temperature for 10 minutes to release 25(OH)D from VDBP and to precipitate proteins. The tubes are centrifuged and supernatant injected onto HPLC-MS/MS. Chromatographic separation involves reverse phase 5 μm, 5 cm × 46 mm, C18 Supelcosil TM analytical column (Bellefonte, PA), and mobile phases: water/0.1% formic acid and methanol/0.1% formic acid. Continuous gradient is used for the separation of 25(OH)D3 and 25(OH)D2. Mass spectrometer is operated in positive ion atmospheric pressure chemical ionization mode. Various multiple reactions monitoring, m/z transitions, are used and optimized for MS/MS analysis. The optimized m/z transitions are listed in **Table 5**. The method has linearity of 1 to 100 ng/mL, and within and between-run imprecision of less than 6%. Ion suppression studies based on internal standard counts in the blank, controls, calibrators, and patient samples showed no

Table 5
Multiple reactions monitoring m/z transitions for 25(OH)D2, 25(OH)D3, and 25(OH)D3 (26, 26, 26, 27, 27, 27-d6)

Analyte	Q1	Q3	Qualifier Ion
25-Hydroxyvitamin D_2	395.5	269.5	377.5
25-Hydroxyvitamin D_3	383.4	257.3	365.5
25-Hydroxyvitamin D_3 (26, 26, 26, 27, 27, 27-d6)	389.3	211.5	263.3

Data from Garg U, Munar A, Frazee C, et al. A simple, rapid atmospheric pressure chemical ionization liquid chromatography tandem mass spectrometry method for the determination of 25-hydroxyvitamin D2 and D3. J Clin Lab Anal 2012;26:349–57.

significant ion suppression. The method was comparable with the solid-phase extraction method used by Mayo and Quest Diagnostics Laboratories. A representative chromatogram is shown in **Fig. 1**.

Note that our published method and most methods described in the literature do not separate 25(OH)D3 from C-3 epimer of 25(OH)D3. Separation of 25(OH)D3 from C-3 epimer of 25(OH)D3 adds a significant analytical run-time and may need a specialized HPLC column. Because levels of C-3 epimer of 25(OH)D3 are low (<5 ng/mL), its presence does not cause any significant problems in most patient samples. However, patients younger than 1 year old may have significant levels of C3-epimer.[24] Stepman and colleagues[25] also showed that even in adults, 3-epimer may be present in significant concentrations and may represent up to 17% of the total 25(OH)D. HPLC-MS/MS methods that can separate C-3 epimer have been described.[24–26]

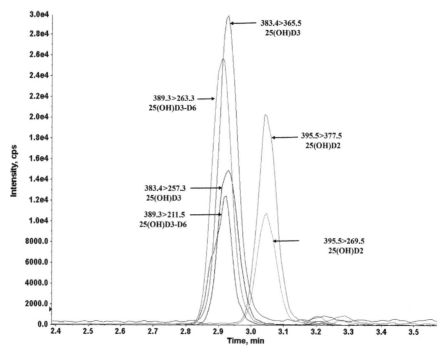

Fig. 1. A representative HPLC-MS/MS chromatogram for 25(OH)D. Different multiple reactions monitoring for 25(OH)D3, 25(OH)D2, and internal standard 25(OH)D3-D6 transitions are shown.

Another inactive metabolite of 25(OH)D, 24,25(OH)D, may also be present in significant concentrations, particularly at high levels of 25(OH)D.[27] Its production is considered a regulatory step in the regulation of 1,25(OH)2D levels, and is stimulated with increasing concentration of 25(OH)D.[27] In HPLC methods, 24,25(OH)D can be chromatographically separated from 25(OH)D and does not cause any interference.

COMPARISON OF IMMUNOASSAYS AND PROTEIN-BINDING ASSAYS WITH CHROMATOGRAPHIC METHODS

Several studies have compared 25(OH)D immunoassays and protein-binding assays with chromatographic methods involving UV detection or mass spectrometry.[15,28–32] Until recently, immunoassays and protein-binding assays suffered from significant inaccuracies and imprecision. Several factors, including inconsistent release of 25(OH)D from VDBP, uneven cross-reactivity of antibody with 25(OH)D3 and 25(OH)D2, interferences from endogenous compounds, and lack of standard materials contributed to these major inaccuracies and imprecision. Over the years, reformulation of reagents and restandardization of immunoassays and protein-binding assays using certified materials have resulted in improved accuracy and precision.[10,11] Despite improvements in 25(OH)D measurement, substantial variability persists among different ligand-based assays. Cross-reactivity with vitamin D metabolites and matrix effects remain an ongoing challenge with these assays. Two potential interfering vitamin D metabolites are 3-epi-25(OH)D3 and 24,25(OH)2D. In DEQAS data, 3-epi-25(OH)D3 showed 56% cross-reactivity in a CPBA but did not show significant cross-reactivity with most antibody-based methods. Cross-reactivity from 24,25(OH)2D, in ligand-binding assays, ranged from less than 5% to 548%.[11] Several studies comparing multiple immunoassays and protein-binding assays with HPLC-UV and HPLC-MS/MS are discussed next.

Farrell and colleagues[31] compared two HPLC-MS/MS and six immunoassays (DiaSorin RIA, Abbott Architect, DiaSorin LIAISON, IDS ISYS, Roche E170, and Siemens Centaur). All immunoassays measured total 25(OH)D, with the exception of the Roche assay, which measured D3 only. The HPLC-MS/MS methods agreed, with a concordance correlation coefficient (CCC) of 0.99 and bias of 0.56 ng/mL. The DiaSorin RIA showed a performance comparable with HPLC-MS/MS, with a CCC of 0.97 and a mean bias of 1.1 ng/mL. Among the immunoassays detecting total 25(OH)D, the CCCs varied between 0.85 (Abbott Architect) to 0.95 (DiaSorin LIAISON). The mean (standard deviation) bias ranged between 0.2 (DiaSorin LIAISON) and 4.56 (Abbott Architect) ng/mL. Most assays demonstrated good intra-assay and interassay precision with Coefficient of Variation less than 10%.

Koivula and colleagues[33] compared four total 25(OH)D automated immunoassays with a commercial (Perkin Elmer) HPLC-MS/MS method using 400 samples collected from a Finnish population. The automated immunoassay methods were DiaSorin Liaison, IDS-iSYS, Abbott ARCHITECT, and Siemens ADVIA Centaur. Mean (95% confidence intervals [CI]) values for these automated methods were 65.6 nmol/L (62.6–68.6), 70.3 nmol/L (67.4–73.1), 69.0 nmol/L (65.5–72.5), and 71.6 nmol/L (68.9–74.3), respectively. Perkin Elmer HPLC-MS/MS mean value was 82.8 nmol/L (79.4–86.2). Differences in the methods were clinically significant. When the reference method (HPLC-MS/MS) gave clinically positive results (over the Finnish reference value $\geq$40 nmol/L) but the immunoassays gave clinically negative results (<40 nmol/L), the results were encoded as false negatives. When the reference method (HPLC-MS/MS) gave clinically negative results (<40 nmol/L) but the immunoassays gave clinically positive results ($\geq$40 nmol/L), the results were encoded as false positives. False-positive numbers by DiaSorin Liaison, IDS-iSYS, Abbott ARCHITECT, and Siemens ADVIA Centaur were 5, 3, 5, and 8 out of 400 samples, respectively. Because the immunoassay gave lower values, the false-negative numbers were even higher: 61, 25, 59, and 22, respectively.

Denimal and colleagues[32] compared seven 25(OH)D immunoassays (two manual and five automated) and three HPLC-UV methods involving different extraction steps with HPLC-MS/MS. Forty-nine human plasma samples with only endogenous 25(OH) D(3) were analyzed with these 11 different methods. The results were analyzed using weighted Deming regression analysis, Bland-Altman plots, and CCC. The results among these assays were comparable with CCC of greater than 90%.

Lippi and colleagues performed a multicenter comparison of seven automated commercial immunoassays: Roche Cobas E601, Beckman Coulter Unicel DXI 800, Ortho Vitros ES, DiaSorin Liaison, Siemens Advia Centaur, Abbott Architect i System and IDS iSYS. Chromsystems Instruments and Chemicals GmbH (Gräfelfing, Germany) HPLC-UV was used as a reference method. A total of 120 outpatient serum samples were prepared, frozen at $-70°C$, and sent frozen to the participating laboratories. The method involves protein precipitation and selective solid phase extraction of 25(OH)D. The data were analyzed using Analyze-it for Deming fit, Spearman correlation, kappa statistical, chi-square test with Yates correction, and Bland-Altman plots. 25(OH)D concentrations in these samples were as follows: median, 78.7 nmol/L; interquartile range, 53.7 to 115 nmol/L; range, 8.2 to 255 nmol/L. Regression coefficients ranged from 0.923 to 0.96, and Deming fit ranged from 0.95 to 1.06. Intercept varied from −15.2 and 9.2 nmol/L, and mean bias varied from −14.5 to 8.7 nmol/L. The minimum performance goal for bias suggested by the Endocrine Society (ie, 15.8%) was slightly exceeded by only one immunoassay (ie, Unicel Dxl −17.1%; 95% CI, −21.7 to −12.4%). Bias of other methods were as follows: Cobas E601, 11.9% (95% CI, −17.2 to −6.5%); Advia Centaur, 11.1% (95% CI, 6.6%–15.6%); Vitros ES, −6.7% (95% CI, −11.9 to −1.5%); Liaison, −5.4% (95% CI, −8.8 to −2.0%); iSYS, 10.7% (95% CI, 7.5%–14.0%); and Architect, 7.9% (95% CI, 4.0%–11.8%). The agreement (kappa statistics) between HPLC and the different immunoassays at the 50 nmol/L 25(OH)D threshold varied between 0.61 and 0.85.

Enko and colleagues, compared IDS-iSYS chemiluminescent immunoassay and ORGENTEC ELISA total 25(OH)D assays with ClinMass HPLC-MS/MS Complete Kit (Waters). The HPLC-MS/MS method separated 25(OH)D2, 25(OH)D3, and C3-epimers. Imprecision of immunoassays at various levels was less than 20%; imprecision of HPLC-MS/MS was less than 10%. In this study, when compared with HPLC-MS/MS, IDS-iSYS and ORGENTEC 25(OH)D assays demonstrated mean relative bias of 16.3% and 17.8%, respectively.

In recent years, manufacturers have reformulated and restandardized their assays with the emphasis on the consistent release of 25(OH)D from VDBP, equimolar recognition of 25(OH)D2 and 25(OH)D3, and assay calibration to certified materials. Despite many improvements, there is a significant variability among different assays, particularly when patients with a broad range of conditions are tested. Heijboer and colleagues[34] investigated the influence of VDBP concentrations on six 25(OH)D assays. Samples were collected from 51 healthy individuals, 52 pregnant women, 50 hemodialysis patients, and 50 intensive care patients. The 25(OH)D methods were Abbot Architect, Siemens Centaur, IDS iSYS, DiaSorin Liaison, Roche Elecsys, DiaSorin RIA, and an ID-XLC-MS/MS. 25(OH)D2 was detected in only 11 out of 203 samples. As expected, pregnant women showed significantly higher, and intensive care patients significantly lower, concentrations of VDBP. Most of the examined 25(OH)D assays showed significant deviations in 25(OH)D concentrations from those of the

ID-XLC-MS/MS method. All methods except Roche Elecsys and DiaSorin RIA showed an inverse relationship between VDBP concentrations and deviations from the ID-XLC-MS/MS results. Annema and colleagues[35] evaluated the new restandardized Abbott Architect 25(OH)D assay in vitamin D–deficient and vitamin D–supplemented individuals. The individuals were given a single dose of 100,000 IU of vitamin D_3. Samples were collected 4 weeks after vitamin D supplementation. As compared with HPLC-MS/MS, Abbott Architect 25(OH)D assay showed a negative bias of 17.4% and 8.9% in vitamin D–insufficient and –supplemented individuals, respectively.

Although HPLC-MS/MS is the gold standard technique for the measurement of 25(OH)D, routine HPLC-MS/MS methods may show inaccuracies and impreci-sion.[10,11,36,37] This is because these instruments are complex; need well-trained personnel; and, in most part, laboratories make their own reagents. Availability of FDA-approved 25(OH)D HPLC-MS/MS kits with premade reagents and calibrators are likely to improve accuracy and precision. Recently, the FDA cleared an HPLC-MS/MS 25(OH)D kit from SCIEX Diagnostics (Framingham, MA). Matrix effects and interferences from vitamin D metabolites may be problematic. Black and col-leagues[37] investigated differences in 25(OH)D concentrations measured at four labo-ratories. Two laboratories used HPLC-MS/MS assays and the third laboratory used the DiaSorin Liaison assay. The fourth laboratory, referred as "certified laboratory," used the HPLC-MS/MS method certified to the standard reference method developed by the NIST and Ghent University. Using Bland-Altman plots, 50 samples were compared in these laboratories. In this comparison, two HPLC-MS/MS methods showed positive bias of 12.4 nmol/L and 12.8 nmol/L as compared with the certified method. The DiaSorin Liaison assay showed a negative bias of 10.6 nmol/L. The prevalence of vitamin D deficiency, as defined by 25(OH) less than 50 nmol/L, was 24%, 16%, 12%, and 41% at the certified laboratory, and laboratories using HPLC-MS/MS methods and DiaSorin Liaison assay.

The studies discussed previously demonstrate that a significant difference remains among different methods of 25(OH)D.

SUMMARY

Vitamin D deficiency has been associated with poor bone health and a myriad of other illnesses including diabetes, cardiovascular diseases, autoimmune disorders, and cancer. Because of these associations and the important role of vitamin D in health and disease, clinical laboratories have seen tremendous growth in 25(OH)D testing in recent years. To classify a patient into a right category of deficiency or sufficiency, accurate measurement of 25(OH)D is of the utmost importance. Although accuracy and precision of 25(OH)D assays have improved overtime, significant differences remain among different methods.

REFERENCES

1. Holick MF. Vitamin D deficiency. N Engl J Med 2007;357:266–81.
2. Holick MF. The vitamin D deficiency pandemic: approaches for diagnosis, treat-ment and prevention. Rev Endocr Metab Disord 2017;18:153–65.
3. LeBlanc ES, Zakher B, Daeges M, et al. Screening for vitamin D deficiency: a sys-tematic review for the U.S. Preventive Services Task Force. Ann Intern Med 2015; 162:109–22.
4. Holick MF, Binkley NC, Bischoff-Ferrari HA, et al. Evaluation, treatment, and pre-vention of vitamin D deficiency: an Endocrine Society clinical practice guideline. J Clin Endocrinol Metab 2011;96:1911–30.

5. Ross AC, Manson JE, Abrams SA, et al. The 2011 report on dietary reference intakes for calcium and vitamin D from the Institute of Medicine: what clinicians need to know. J Clin Endocrinol Metab 2011;96:53–8.

6. Srivastava T, Garg U, Ruiz M, et al. Serum 25(OH)-vitamin D level in children: is there a need to change the reference range based on 2011 Institute of Medicine report? Clin Pediatr (Phila) 2013;52:178–82.

7. Ross AC. The 2011 report on dietary reference intakes for calcium and vitamin D. Public Health Nutr 2011;14:938–9.

8. Pludowski P, Karczmarewicz E, Bayer M, et al. Practical guidelines for the supplementation of vitamin D and the treatment of deficits in Central Europe: recommended vitamin D intakes in the general population and groups at risk of vitamin D deficiency. Endokrynol Pol 2013;64:319–27.

9. Okazaki R, Ozono K, Fukumoto S, et al. Assessment criteria for vitamin D deficiency/insufficiency in Japan: proposal by an expert panel supported by Research Program of Intractable Diseases, Ministry of Health, Labour and Welfare, Japan, The Japanese Society for Bone and Mineral Research and The Japan Endocrine Society [Opinion]. Endocr J 2017;64:1–6.

10. Carter GD, Berry J, Durazo-Arvizu R, et al. Hydroxyvitamin D assays: an historical perspective from DEQAS. J Steroid Biochem Mol Biol 2018;177:30–5.

11. Carter GD, Jones JC, Shannon J, et al. 25-Hydroxyvitamin D assays: potential interference from other circulating vitamin D metabolites. J Steroid Biochem Mol Biol 2016;164:134–8.

12. Le Goff C, Cavalier E, Souberbielle JC, et al. Measurement of circulating 25-hydroxyvitamin D: a historical review. Pract Lab Med 2015;2:1–14.

13. Hollis BW, Kamerud JQ, Selvaag SR, et al. Determination of vitamin D status by radioimmunoassay with an 125I-labeled tracer. Clin Chem 1993;39:529–33.

14. Lensmeyer GL, Wiebe DA, Binkley N, et al. HPLC method for 25-hydroxyvitamin D measurement: comparison with contemporary assays. Clin Chem 2006;52:1120–6.

15. Carrozza C, Persichilli S, Canu G, et al. Measurement of 25-hydroxyvitamin vitamin D by liquid chromatography tandem-mass spectrometry with comparison to automated immunoassays. Clin Chem Lab Med 2012;50:2033–5.

16. Garg U, Munar A, Frazee C 3rd, et al. A simple, rapid atmospheric pressure chemical ionization liquid chromatography tandem mass spectrometry method for the determination of 25-hydroxyvitamin D2 and D3. J Clin Lab Anal 2012; 26:349–57.

17. Jones G, Kaufmann M. Vitamin D metabolite profiling using liquid chromatography-tandem mass spectrometry (LC-MS/MS). J Steroid Biochem Mol Biol 2016;164: 110–4.

18. Jumaah F, Larsson S, Essen S, et al. A rapid method for the separation of vitamin D and its metabolites by ultra-high performance supercritical fluid chromatography-mass spectrometry. J Chromatogr A 2016;1440:191–200.

19. Lee S, Kim JH, Kim SA, et al. A rapid and simple liquid-chromatography-tandem mass spectrometry method for measuring 25-hydroxyvitamin d2 and 25-hydroxyvitamin d3 in human serum: comparison with two automated immunoassays. Ann Clin Lab Sci 2016;46:645–53.

20. Mineva EM, Schleicher RL, Chaudhary-Webb M, et al. A candidate reference measurement procedure for quantifying serum concentrations of 25-hydroxyvitamin D(3) and 25-hydroxyvitamin D(2) using isotope-dilution liquid chromatography-tandem mass spectrometry. Anal Bioanal Chem 2015;407:5615–24.

21. Singh RJ. Quantitation of 25-OH-vitamin D (25OHD) using liquid tandem mass spectrometry (LC-MS-MS). Methods Mol Biol 2010;603:509–17.

22. van den Ouweland JM, Beijers AM, Demacker PN, et al. Measurement of 25-OH-vitamin D in human serum using liquid chromatography tandem-mass spectrometry with comparison to radioimmunoassay and automated immunoassay. J Chromatogr B Analyt Technol Biomed Life Sci 2010;878:1163–8.

23. van den Ouweland JM, Vogeser M, Bacher S. Vitamin D and metabolites measurement by tandem mass spectrometry. Rev Endocr Metab Disord 2013;14:159–84.

24. Singh RJ, Taylor RL, Reddy GS, et al. C-3 epimers can account for a significant proportion of total circulating 25-hydroxyvitamin D in infants, complicating accurate measurement and interpretation of vitamin D status. J Clin Endocrinol Metab 2006;91:3055–61.

25. Stepman HC, Vanderroost A, Stockl D, et al. Full-scan mass spectral evidence for 3-epi-25-hydroxyvitamin D(3) in serum of infants and adults. Clin Chem Lab Med 2011;49:253–6.

26. Bailey D, Veljkovic K, Yazdanpanah M, et al. Analytical measurement and clinical relevance of vitamin D(3) C3-epimer. Clin Biochem 2013;46:190–6.

27. Cashman KD, Hayes A, Galvin K, et al. Significance of serum 24,25-dihydroxyvitamin D in the assessment of vitamin D status: a double-edged sword? Clin Chem 2015;61:636–45.

28. Koivula MK, Turpeinen U, Laitinen P, et al. Comparison of automated 25-OH vitamin D immunoassays with liquid chromatography isotope dilution tandem mass spectrometry. Clin Lab 2012;58:1253–61.

29. Kocak FE, Ozturk B, Isiklar OO, et al. A comparison between two different automated total 25-hydroxyvitamin D immunoassay methods using liquid chromatography-tandem mass spectrometry. Biochem Med (Zagreb) 2015;25:430–8.

30. Kelley JM, Melanson SE, Snyder ML, et al. Method comparison of a 25-hydroxy vitamin D enzyme immunoassay to liquid chromatography tandem mass spectroscopy. Clin Chem Lab Med 2012;50:1137–8.

31. Farrell CJ, Martin S, McWhinney B, et al. State-of-the-art vitamin D assays: a comparison of automated immunoassays with liquid chromatography-tandem mass spectrometry methods. Clin Chem 2012;58:531–42.

32. Denimal D, Ducros V, Dupre T, et al. Agreement of seven 25-hydroxy vitamin D(3) immunoassays and three high performance liquid chromatography methods with liquid chromatography tandem mass spectrometry. Clin Chem Lab Med 2014;52:511–20.

33. Koivula MK, Matinlassi N, Laitinen P, et al. Four automated 25-OH total vitamin D immunoassays and commercial liquid chromatography tandem-mass spectrometry in Finnish population. Clin Lab 2013;59:397–405.

34. Heijboer AC, Blankenstein MA, Kema IP, et al. Accuracy of 6 routine 25-hydroxyvitamin D assays: influence of vitamin D binding protein concentration. Clin Chem 2012;58:543–8.

35. Annema W, Nowak A, von Eckardstein A, et al. Evaluation of the new restandardized Abbott Architect 25-OH Vitamin D assay in vitamin D-insufficient and vitamin D-supplemented individuals. J Clin Lab Anal 2018;32(4):e22328.

36. Couchman L, Benton CM, Moniz CF. Variability in the analysis of 25-hydroxyvitamin D by liquid chromatography-tandem mass spectrometry: the devil is in the detail. Clin Chim Acta 2012;413:1239–43.

37. Black LJ, Anderson D, Clarke MW, et al. Analytical bias in the measurement of serum 25-hydroxyvitamin D concentrations impairs assessment of vitamin D status in clinical and research settings. PLoS One 2015;10:e0135478.

Pain Management Testing by Liquid Chromatography Tandem Mass Spectrometry

Geza S. Bodor, MD

KEYWORDS

- Opiates • Opioids • Pain medication • LC-MSMS • Liquid chromatography
- Tandem mass spectrometry

KEY POINTS

- Opioid pain medications cause severe social and financial burden because of their severe side effects.
- Addiction prevention requires accurate and sensitive testing for monitoring patient compliance with prescriptions.
- Testing must include opiates, synthetic opioids, illicit drugs, and prescription drugs with abuse potential.
- The commercially available opiate immunoassays cannot fulfill the requirements of pain medication monitoring.
- Liquid chromatography tandem mass spectrometry methods are ideal for pain medication monitoring, but require careful method development, validation, and result interpretation.

INTRODUCTION

Opioids, chemicals that bind to tissue opioid receptors, have gained much attention in recent years owing to their increasing impact on public and individual's health. Opioid prescribing trends have been increasing from 1999 through 2016, the last year for which complete statistics are available, bringing with it the unprecedented increase in opioid overdoses and related deaths.[1] By the end of 2015, 63% of all drug overdose-related deaths were due to opioids, surpassing 33,000 lethal cases that year. The highest number of deaths were due to fentanyl and its analogs (20,100 deaths), followed by heroin and prescription opioids (15,400 and 14,400 deaths, respectively). The number of opioid related deaths has surpassed that of cocaine or

Disclosure Statement: Nothing to disclose.
Department of Pathology, University of Colorado Anschutz Medical Campus, University of Colorado, Leprino Building, Room 229, Mail Stop A022, 12401 East 17th Avenue, Aurora, CO 80045, USA
E-mail address: geza.bodor@ucdenver.edu

methamphetamine[1,2] and exceeded that of deaths related to human immunodeficiency virus infection in its peak year.

This increase is largely due to opioid use to alleviation of chronic, nonmalignant pain, in contrast with earlier practice of opioid use at the end of life and for malignant pain treatment. The proportion of visits to medical providers for nonmalignant pain has shown an approximately 26% increase in the United States from 2000 to 2010. The proportion of visits with provider-diagnosed pain has increased by approximately 50%,[3] whereas the proportion of visits when opioids were prescribed more than doubled.[3]

The economic burden to US society was estimated to be $78 billion in 2013,[4] but the revised cost by The Council of Economic Advisers projected $500 billion just 2 years later.[5] This substantial increase is attributed to the increasing number of opioid overdose-related cases within the time the studies were conducted and to the fact that the paper by Florence and colleagues[4] only calculated health care-related cost, whereas the report by the Council of Economic Advisers estimated all cost to society. Regardless of accounting practices, the opioid epidemic is a serious burden on US society and must be dealt with. For successful intervention, appropriate tools must be applied before remedies can be offered to the individual and the community.

THE NEED FOR OPIOID TESTING

Opioids are very effective pain killers, but have side effects ranging from nausea, vomiting, and miosis to coma or severe respiratory depression, leading to death. Uncommon side effects include confusion, hallucinations, delirium, muscle rigidity, myoclonus, and opioid-induced hyperalgesia during cessation of drug administration.

The most severe side effects—namely, tolerance, dependence, and addiction—belong to the group of reinforcement disorders. Tolerance, which requires successively larger doses of the drug to achieve the same medical effect, can develop with even short-term opioid use. Tolerance can be also lost when the patient has no access to opioids for a while, as during incarceration. Regaining access to opioids again, the person restarts his or her drug intake at the previous doses and the lost tolerance leads to a severe outcome.[6,7] Dependence, a change in the individual's metabolism, forces the patient to continue use of the drugs beyond the cessation of pain. Addiction, the most severe side effect of opioid use, is composed of physiologic and behavioral changes that lead to drug-seeking behavior, often via criminal means. The side effects of withdrawal force the patient back to repeat drug use, or when prescription is no longer available, to obtain the opioid via illegal means.

The combination of tolerance, dependence, and addiction can turn the patient toward readily available illicit opioids such as heroin, illegal versions of the prescription drugs such black market methadone or fentanyl, or designer opioids such fentanyl analogs or Krokodil (desomorphine). Diverting legally obtained opioids, that is, selling the prescription medication on the streets is another aberrant behavior that is often associated with sample adulteration in the form of "spiking" the sample with the prescribed drug to mask lack of use.

Patients on chronic opioid therapy are required to sign a medical agreement or contract that stipulates conditions for participation in the treatment. By signing, the patient agrees that all controlled substances come from prescription by a medical provider; the patient will inform the prescriber of any change in his or her medication, health status, or the presence of side effects; that he or she will not share or allow the use of his or her medication by another person; and he or she submits to random urine drug tests.

The study by Michna and colleagues[8] has found that only 55% of 470 patients on chronic pain treatment were compliant, despite the strict regulations. Approximately 10% were missing their prescribed medication, 14.5% had other opioids that could not be explained by prescription and metabolism, and 20% had illicit drugs. The study by Couto and colleagues[9] found, in a retrospective study, that results from 938,000 samples indicated that approximately 75% of the patients were being non-compliant: 38% had no detectable concertation of the prescribed drug, 29% had nonprescribed medication, and 11% had illicit drugs in their system. An additional 32% showed drug concentrations that were inconsistent with the dose they were taking. The percentages add up to more than 100% because a patient may fall into more than 1 category.

Because of the high proportion of patients on opioids use unprescribed and illicit drugs, pain medication testing customarily includes monitoring of prescription and illicit drugs in addition to various opiates and synthetic opioids in the test panel.

METABOLISM AND CHEMICAL DIVERSITY OF OPIOIDS

All opioids act as agonists or antagonists on the body's opioid receptors, but the physiologic similarity does not depend on chemical similarities of all opioids. There are 4 major classes of opioids: phenanthrenes, benzomorphans, phenylpiperidines, and diphenylheptanes (**Fig. 1**) and each class contains multiple chemicals.

Most of the opioid analgesics are alkaloids of the poppy plant (*Papaver somniferum*) or derivatives of these natural compounds. Morphine and codeine belong to the phenanthrene class of chemicals and are known as opiates or natural opiates. Chemical modifications of the natural opiates create the semisynthetic opiates. Several semisynthetic opiates are prescription drugs (**Table 1**), but can also be metabolites of other semisynthetic opiates (**Fig. 2**). They are eliminated via phase I deactivation and phase II conjugation to glucuronic acid at the 3 or 6 carbon atoms before being excreted in the urine. For a comprehensive review of opioid metabolism see Smith.[10]

Because natural and synthetic opioids undergo extensive phase I metabolism via the CYP enzyme system and phase II metabolism by glucuronide conjugation before excretion, inherited genetic factors, coadministration of other drugs, age, sex, and liver and kidney disease may influence the speed of metabolism and the number of metabolites detectable at a given time. The presence of a particular opiate could be the sign of compliance with prescriptions or use of nonprescribed medication or illicit narcotics. In contrast, the absence of the prescribed drug could mean noncompliance or diversion, but could also be due to metabolism of the parent drug. Accurate assessment of the patient's compliance requires analytical methods of high analytical specificity and sensitivity, as well as expert interpretation of results.

Opioids that belong to the benzomorphan, phenylpiperidine, or diphenylheptane groups are synthetic opioids. Their chemical structure is significantly different from that of opiates and, thus, may not be detected by common laboratory methods. Their metabolism is unique (**Table 2**) and it produces characteristic metabolites that are different from those of opiates.

Patients with addiction disorders often will consume multiple drugs, including non-opioid prescription medications such as benzodiazepines, or will abuse illicit drugs such as cocaine, marijuana, or amphetamines. If consumption of unauthorized drug is detected, the patient could be disqualified from further treatment with narcotic

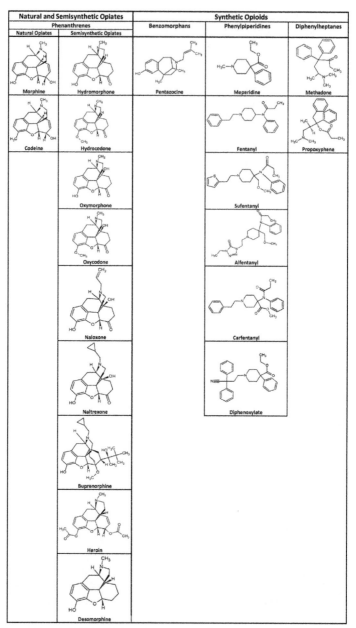

Fig. 1. Chemical structure of opiates and opioids. Opiates and opioids are listed by chemical class of their main structure.

analgesics; therefore, the monitoring of drugs of abuse along with opioids is common practice. The chemical structure of drugs with abuse potential is dissimilar to opiates and opioids; therefore, they require alternative monitoring—either a combination of a large number of specific immunoassays or the use of a chromatography mass spectrometry–based panel.

Table 1
Prescription narcotic analgesic opioids

Chemical Class	Generic Name	Brand Names	Notes
Phenantrenes			
Opiates (natural)	Morphine	Arymo ER, Duramorph, Infumorph P/F, MorphaBond ER, MS Contin	Available under its generic name also
	Codeine	Calcidrine, Colrex, Phenflu, Rolatuss, Tylenol with Codeine #3 or #4	Available under its generic name also
Opiates (semisynthetic)	Hydromorphone	Dilaudid	Available under its generic name also
	Hydrocodone	Anexsia, Dicodid, Hycodan, Hycomine, Lorcet, Lortab, Norco, Tussionex, Vicodin	Available under its generic name also
	Oxymorphone	Opana	Available under its generic name also
	Oxycodone	OxyContin, Percodan, Percocet	Available under its generic name also
	Naloxone	Narcan, Talwin NX (with pentazocine), Suboxone (with buprenorphine)	Available under its generic name also
	Naltrexone	Revia, Vivitrol	
	Buprenorphine	Suboxone (with naloxone)	Available under its generic name also
	Heroin		Illegal drug
	Desomorphine		Illegal drug ('Krokodil')
Synthetic opioids			
Benzomorphans	Pentazocine	Fortral, Fortwin, Sosegon, Talacen, Talwin, Talwin NX (with naloxone)	
Phenylpiperidines	Meperidine	Demerol	Available under its generic name also
	Fentanyl	Duragesic, Sublimaze, Subsys	Available under its generic name also
	Sufentanil	Sufenta	
	Alfentanil	Alfenta, Rapifen	
	Carfentanil	Wildnil	Illegal drug. Veterinary use
	Diphenoxylate	Lomotil, Lonox, Lomanate	
Diphenylheptanes	Methadone	Dolophine	Available under its generic name also
	Propoxyphene	Darvon, Dolane	Available under its generic name also

SAMPLE SELECTION FOR PAIN MEDICATION TESTING

Workplace drug testing has been using urine as the sample of choice for decades and this practice was also adopted for pain medication testing. Urine is available in large quantity, it can contain the parent drug as well as the metabolites in relatively high concentration, and multiple sample preparation methods are available (discussed elsewhere in this article). Urine can also act as a "reservoir," allowing the detection of

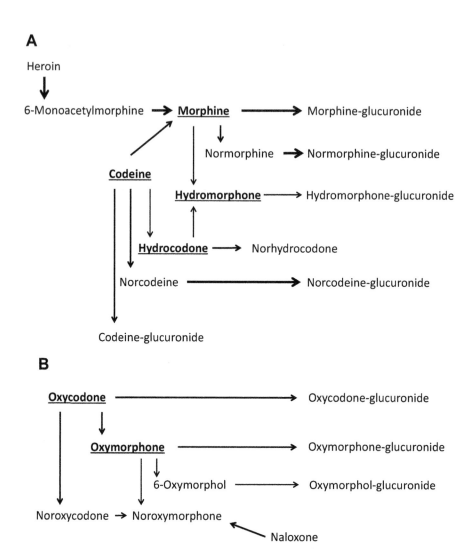

Fig. 2. Metabolism of opiates. Only analytically and medically significant metabolites of natural and semisynthetic opiates are presented with their metabolic pathways. Minor metabolites have been omitted for clarity. Opiates available as prescription drugs are printed in bold and underlined. (*A*) Metabolic pathways involving morphine, codeine, hydromorphone and hydrocodone. (*B*) Metabolism of oxycodone.

drug use longer than could be expected based on the drug's half-life. Urine is a suitable sample for both immunoassays and liquid chromatography tandem mass spectrometry (LC-MSMS) methods. Disadvantages of urine as the analytical sample are ease of adulteration or substitution, the possibility that the patient will not be able to produce a sample at the time of demand, and the wide concentration range of physiologic contents that might compromise analyte recovery of the drug of interest. Because of the extensive glucuronide conjugation of opioids during phase II metabolism, free (unconjugated) and conjugated drugs are present simultaneously, requiring either separate measurement of free and conjugated analytes or hydrolysis

Table 2
Metabolites of synthetic opioids

Synthetic Opioids	Metabolites
Pentazocine	Pentazocine-glucuronide
Meperidine	Normeperidine
Fentanyl	Norfentanyl
Sufentanil	Norsufentanil, methylsufentanil
Alfentanil	Noralfentanil, phenylpropionamide
Carfentanil	Norcarfentanil
Diphenoxylate	Difenoxin
Propoxyphene	Norpropoxyphene (m/z 326), dehydrated rearrangement product (m/z 308)
Methadone	EDDP (2-ethylidene-1,5-dimethyl-3,3-diphenylpyrrolidine), EMDP (2-ethyl-5methyl-3,3-diphenyl-1-pyrroline)
Buprenorphine	Norbuprenorphine

Minor and unconfirmed metabolites are not listed.

treatment of the sample. Furthermore, urine drug concentrations are not correlated with simultaneously observed blood concentration; therefore, accurate conclusions regarding dosing cannot be provided from a urine result.

Saliva has been used as the sample for pain management testing purposes relatively recently because of the 1 to 2 orders of magnitude lower drug concentration in saliva than in urine. These concentrations are below the detectable concentrations of many immunoassays. With the introduction of LC-MSMS into clinical laboratory testing saliva has become a viable sample and multiple LC-MSMS–based methods have been published in the literature for salivary opioid testing,[11–15] but the multitude of collection devices complicates saliva testing. These devices are not equivalent in their buffer composition, preservative content, and other properties that can introduce matrix effects in LC-MSMS testing; therefore, the validation of acceptable collection devices is mandatory and samples should only be accepted for testing if they arrive in an approved device. The advantages of saliva testing include ease of collection and easy observation of the patient during collection to prevent adulteration. Salivary drug concentration better correlates with blood drug concentrations than does that of urine.

Blood, serum, or plasma may be also used for pain medication testing, but have special characteristics. The most important of these characteristics is the influence of the parent drug's half-life on the number of detectable analytes. Short-acting opioids such as fentanyl (half-life of 3.5–4.0 hours) may not be detected in blood, serum, or plasma after 1 day after administration via injection, but administration via transdermal patch will produce detection times of several days or weeks. Taking opioid metabolism into consideration during pain medication result interpretation is even more important when blood, serum, or plasma is used versus urine result interpretation. Among the other negative aspects of using blood, serum, or plasma is the need for venipuncture and possible sample processing at the collection site. If plasma is used, the anticoagulant might introduce matrix effects with LC-MSMS methods and, therefore, the acceptable anticoagulants must be evaluated during method validation and explicitly stated in the instructions to providers. Positive attributes of blood testing are the correlation of blood opioid concentration to dosing and time of last dose; however, reported blood opioid concentrations have shown extreme values in tolerant individuals as compared with opioid-naïve patients.[16,17] The exceptionally high blood opioid concentrations might suggest interference, but the presence of the appropriate metabolites would substantiate adherence to prescriptions.

ANALYSIS OF OPIOIDS
Immunoassays

Immunoassays have become the mainstay of pain medication testing since the 1970s when the Department of Defense started drug testing of soldiers returning from Vietnam. In response to the heroin epidemic of that time, morphine and codeine became the targets for opiate drug testing. The immunoassays were designed to report results qualitatively as positive if the morphine or codeine concentration exceeded a predetermined cutoff or result it as negative otherwise. Relatively high cutoff concentrations were established to compensate for the shortcomings of the early analytical methods and to comply with the assumption of innocence principle of the law. Heroin testing in the form of detection of heroin metabolite 6-monoacetyl morphine later became part of the opiate testing protocol. The 2 opiates, morphine and codeine, as well as 6-monoacetyl morphine, remain the designated targets of opiate immunoassays and assay cutoffs are regulated only for them, but not for the other semisynthetic opiates or synthetic opioids. Because of the chemical similarities between natural and semisynthetic opiates (see **Fig. 1**), these assays will show some degree of cross-reactivity with other compounds than morphine or codeine, but the limit of detection will vary depending on the brand of assay and the actual opiate present.[18] Bertholf and colleagues[19] presented evidence recently showing that immunoassays calibrated to 300 ng/mL morphine are inadequate for monitoring relatively strongly cross reacting opiates such as hydrocodone and hydromorphone. The immunoassay, calibrated to give positive result at 300 ng/mL morphine concentration, deemed negative 72% of the 112 urine samples containing 1 or both of these drugs at concentrations of greater than 50 ng/mL. Nineteen percent of the samples contained hydrocodone or hydromorphone of greater than 300 ng/mL and an additional 28% of the samples the sum of the concentrations of these drugs were greater than 300 ng/mL. When multiple types of opiates are present, they can react additively to generate a positive immunoassay response, even when the concentration of each of the cross-reacting opiates is below the cutoff. Immunoassays are class, not drug, specific; therefore, the identity of simultaneously consumed narcotics cannot be verified by an immunoassay. The presence of an unprescribed drug could be mistaken for compliance. In conclusion, immunoassays are inadequate for the assessment of compliance. Many semisynthetic opiates but none of the synthetic opioids are detected by the morphine–codeine opiate immunoassays, although specialized immunoassays have been developed to detect common semisynthetic opiates such as oxymorphone or buprenorphine, or synthetic ones as methadone or fentanyl.

Immunoassay cutoffs, established to satisfy legal standards, have insufficient sensitivity for pain monitoring. Higher cutoffs lead to significantly lower detection rates.[20] The false-negative result, when the patient is on low-dose medication, would mistakenly accuse the patient of diverting his prescription. The 2-step, screening–confirmation, drug testing policy does prevent false-negative reports, because screen-negative samples are not commonly sent for follow-up testing (selection bias). To prevent mistaken exclusion of patients from necessary treatment, pain medication testing must use as low a limit of detection as possible from an analytical method of high selectivity, and the appropriate assays must report actual measured concentration for the drugs found in the sample.

Chromatography-mass spectrometry-based pain medication analysis
Chromatography-mass spectrometry methods can provide the necessary sensitivity and selectivity for accurate pain medication testing. Numerous LC-MSMS methods have been published in the medical literature, in trade publications from chromatography column and high-pressure liquid chromatography (HPLC) or mass spectrometer manufacturers. Many of these methods present chromatograms of pure analytical substances in solvents, but they might not work in real-life applications using biological samples in various matrices. Additional difficulty is encountered when pain panels, containing several dozens of drugs (**Box 1**), are used for pain medication testing. Differences in concentrations, chromatographic separation, ease of ionization, and fragmentation are independent variables, requiring source and compound specific parameters to be optimized simultaneously for each drug in the panel. Unsatisfactory optimization might not be recognized until method validation, necessitating the return to method development again. A detailed discussion of LC-MSMS method development is not possible within the scope of this article. For the interested laboratory scientist, there are excellent training courses in LC-MSMS method development and validation offered by the Association for Mass Spectrometry: Applications to the Clinical Lab and the American Association for Clinical Chemistry.

Sample preparation for liquid chromatography tandem mass spectrometry testing
The simplest sample preparation for urine is the "dilute and shoot" method, where an aliquot of the patient's sample is mixed with a buffer and the internal standard then this mixture is injected in the LC-MSMS. For saliva and blood, this simple sample preparation might not be sufficient. The low concentration of analytes in these samples often requires cell lysis, protein precipitation, and removal of phospholipids before analysis can be attempted. Initial liquid–liquid extraction, followed by evaporation, concentration, and reconstitution in the injection buffer or solvent is a common sample preparation process. Solid phase extraction is another commonly applied sample preparation step using single solid phase extraction columns or microtiter plates. The preparation method used depends on the analyte to be measured, number of samples tested per run, and the availability of sample handling (robotic) pipetting station. Appropriately equipped HPLCs can be programmed to perform in-line sample extraction or purification.

Box 1
Drug classes that are commonly measured by liquid chromatography tandem mass spectrometry in pain panels

Amphetamines

Barbiturates

Benzodiazepines

Cannabinoids

Cocaine, benzoylecgonine

Muscle relaxants (eg, carisoprodol)

Opiates (natural and semisynthetic)

Opioids

Phencyclidine

Benzodiazepines and opioids can be excreted in the urine as free drugs or be conjugated to glucuronide or sulfates and the ratio of free to conjugated opioids might depend on the patient's renal function.[21] Glucuronide-conjugated drugs may be present at similar or greater concentrations in urine than the free drugs; therefore, the laboratory must decide if they want to measure free or total (free + conjugated) concentrations.[22,23] Conjugated drugs may be separated chromatographically and measured directly by the mass spectrometer.[24] If measurement of total drugs is desired, the sample must be hydrolyzed by acids or glucuronidase enzyme. Several hydrolysis methods have been published, but they are not equivalent in efficiency depending on the source of the glucuronidase enzyme and the type of opioid.[25]

Acid hydrolysis was reported to be more efficient removing glucuronide than enzymes, but buprenorphine and its metabolite, norbuprenorphine, were resistant to acid hydrolysis.[26,27] If enzymatic hydrolysis is applied, sample extraction must follow to remove the high concentration of added protein from the urine sample before analysis. Incomplete hydrolysis is an unwelcome complication of enzymatic treatment; therefore, the method must be optimized during development and hydrolysis efficiency must be carefully monitored with appropriate quality control samples.

Overview of liquid chromatography tandem mass spectrometry methods

Many types of reversed phase columns, such as C-18, biphenyl, or phenyl-hexyl, have all been used for the chromatographic separation of opioids and other monitored drugs. Mobile phases of water, methanol, and acetonitrile are most commonly used in a gradient elution scheme. Proper chromatographic conditions allow the separation of 30 to 100 drugs in less than 10 minutes injection-to-injection times. Longer chromatography, although advantageous for separating interferences from the analyte(s) of interest, can compromise throughput. HPLC and ultra-high pressure liquid chromatography (UHPLC) differ in column and resin bead size, the amount of mobile phase and sample volume needed for the run, and the pressure they operate under. HPLC typically works at less than 5000 psi, but UHPLC operates up to 7000 to 15,000 psi depending on the pump and column. The increased pressure allows faster separation, but UHPLC has its own special method development considerations.[28]

Most drugs monitored in pain medication testing will ionize either by electrospray or atmospheric pressure chemical ionization, and both of these methods have been used for drug testing by LC-MSMS. In tandem mass spectrometry analysis, the analyte of interest is selected by its mass-to-charge ratio (m/z) in the first quadrupole and then it is fragmented before the fragments can be analyzed in the third quadrupole. The parent ion and fragments, or daughter ions, are distinctive for the drug and provide positive identification beyond the chromatographic retention time. A pair of parent/daughter ions, called a transition, is monitored but, for high-fidelity drug identification, at least 2 transitions must be monitored per analyte and at least 1 transition per internal standard. Special circumstances may dictate monitoring of more transitions. The parameters driving the quadrupoles and the collision energy, the compound specific parameters, must be individually optimized for each analyte and each fragment during method development and might have to be revised during initial method validation.

Wide analytical measurement range is another requirement in pain medication testing because of the more than 3 orders of magnitude difference in drug concentration often seen with opioid use. The method must be robust enough not to exhibit a hook effect at extremely high concentrations, and column and detector saturation must be recognized by the operator if accurate quantitation is required at the high end of the concentration range.

With large pain panels containing several dozen drugs and metabolites, monitoring 2 or 3 transitions per drug for the duration of the run might not be practical. If instrument capacity is divided between many transitions, sensitivity and peak resolution could suffer owing to too short a dwell time. To prevent this, modern mass spectrometers can be programmed to acquire fewer transitions for a limited period of time around the expected retention time of an analyte then switch to a different set of transitions. This mode is called scheduled multiple reaction monitoring. Scheduled multiple reaction monitoring is necessary for large panels of pain medication testing and allows for the quantitative analysis of 50 to 100 analytes in the same run or qualitative analysis of even more.

Several LC-MSMS methods have been described in the literature for the monitoring of patients on pain medication[29–32] and even more unpublished reports are used in various laboratories as laboratory developed tests. The published pain medication methods usually focus on the opioid drugs and their metabolites, but often include other prescription and illicit drugs as well (see **Box 1**). The published panels can detect as few as 20 but sometimes as many as more than 100 drugs and metabolites simultaneously within a few minutes per sample. Instrument and chromatography column manufacturers have also described methods for pain panel testing as application notes for their columns, but many of these methods are proof of concept because they lack any data on method validation using clinical samples.

The traditional separation methods use reversed phase chromatography on C-18 columns but more recently new separation chemistries have been also described using pentafluorophenyl[29] or phenylhexyl[31] columns. The lower limit of quantitation varies between less than 1 ng/mL and up to 100 ng/mL, depending on the analyte and its clinically relevant concentration range. Some commercial laboratories have calibrated their LC-MSMS assays at even higher cutoff concentrations to conform to workplace drug testing standards, but higher detection limits will produce more false-negative results.[33] A recent study by Krock and colleagues[34] investigated the impact of lowering the detection limit of drugs in an LC-MSMS pain panel and found that lowering the cutoff concentration by 1 order of magnitude will increase sensitivity of detection by 10% to 20%. Clonazepam, benzoylecgonine, hydromorphone, and fentanyl produced a 94%, 45%, 37%, and 32% higher detection proportion, respectively, at the lower cutoffs.

The type of mass spectrometer most often used for quantitative analysis is the triple-quadrupole instrument, but other methods using ion trap[35,36] have also been published. Up to a 30-fold increase in the signal-to-noise ratio of the ion trap method over traditional full scan methods allows lower drug detection limits.[35] Other hybrid mass spectrometric methods using time of flight and triple quadruple mass spectrometers have also been described[37] for quantitative analysis, but time of flight or other types of accurate mass instruments are most commonly applied to drug screening.

Synthetic opioids are another group of pain medications that have their own special requirements for analysis. The primary route of metabolism for synthetic opioids is N-demethylation, which forms nor-metabolites and the nor-metabolites usually have longer half-lives than the parent drugs. The nor-metabolites, therefore, can accumulate in the body and can be detected for a longer period of time than their parents. It is not uncommon for synthetic opioid metabolites to be detected days after the parent drug's concentration has decreased below assay detection limits; therefore, pain medication panels should test for the nor-metabolites of buprenorphine, fentanyl, meperidine, methadone, and propoxyphene. The study by DePriest and colleagues[38] found the ratio of samples that contained the nor-metabolites of these opioids to be between 8% and 53% and the detection rate of synthetic opioids increased between 9% and 113% when metabolites were included in addition to the parent drug.

The effects of isobaric compounds on liquid chromatography tandem mass spectrometry methods

Isobaric opioids (**Box 2**) have the same parent ion m/z ratios and they often fragment into the same daughter ions as well; therefore, they cannot be distinguished from each other by their transitions. Isobaric compounds must be separated chromatographically and the retention time (RT) of the isobaric compounds must allow for completion of acquisition of 1 peak before the peak of the next isobaric drug starts eluting. This requires very careful chromatography method design and extensive validation.[39,40] When more than 2 isobaric compounds might be present in a sample, the chromatography run should be extended to prevent cross-talk between the different drugs.

Matrix effects

Biological matrices such as urine, saliva, and blood can contain salts, proteins, cellular material, lipids, and other small molecules at large between-individual concentration variations. They may contain biological contaminants that are normally not components of that matrix, such as blood or bacteria in urine, during disease. The presence of these unknown substances can have undesirable effects on mass spectrometric analysis via ion suppression or ion enhancement; therefore, method validation focused on matrix effects are mandatory and now required by Clinical and Laboratory Standards Institute and College of American Pathologists (CAP) standards.[41] Matrix effect studies to assess ion suppression or enhancement can be done using sample mixing studies or flow injection through a T-connector, where effluent from the HPLC is mixed with a low concentration of the analyte from a syringe pump.[42,43] The change in analyte signal intensity versus baseline signal intensity around the peak of interest provides the measure of ion suppression if present. Ion suppression of less than 20% could be compensated by the use of stable isotope internal standard of the same composition as the analyte, but not all analytes are available in deuterated or carbon isotope variants. If an appropriate internal standard is not available or the ion suppression or enhancement is greater than approximately 20%, an alternate sample cleanup procedure or alternate chromatography conditions must be developed.[43]

RESULT REPORTING AND INTERPRETATION

LC-MSMS testing of patients on chronic pain medication provides a large amount of data that can overwhelm the clinician. LC-MSMS is capable of reporting the presence

---

Box 2
Isobaric opioids

Morphine (285.34), hydromorphone (285.34), norcodeine (285.34), norhydrocodone (285.34), pentazocine (285.43)

Codeine (299.37), hydrocodone (299.37)

Oxymorphone (301.34), dihydrocodeine (301.39)

Normorphine (271.32), norhydromorphone (271.32), desmorphine (271.36)

Naloxone (327.38), 6-Monoacetyl-morphine (327.38)

Molecular weights are given in parenthesis for each compound, rounded to 2 decimal places.

or absence of parent drugs and multiple metabolites as well as their concentrations. Pain panels are not standardized with regard to analytes and cutoff or lower limit of quantitation concentrations; therefore, the clinician needs help in selecting the appropriate test(s) to answer the most important clinical question: Is the patient compliant with the prerequisites for obtaining the prescription? When the result is returned from the laboratory, the clinician also might require expert help for correct interpretation of those results. Correct interpretation, in turn, requires adequate knowledge of pharmacokinetics of opioid metabolism or that of other drugs being monitored. Laboratory testing of pain medications does not start or end with analysis of the samples. Multiple studies have shown that physicians can have difficulty in understanding and interpreting the drug test's results, even when they routinely prescribe those medications.[44–48] This lack of knowledge extends through multiple disciplines and includes pain physicians, too.

The presence of drugs and metabolites depends on dosing regimen and timing of sample collection to last dose of the drug; therefore, interpretation must be interdisciplinary. The laboratory director has the responsibility for informing the clinician of the significance and possible meaning of the results, but the clinician must also provide the necessary information to the laboratory. Collaboration and open communication between the laboratory and the clinician is absolutely mandatory for proper application of pain management testing in clinical practice if we want to provide the best clinical care to our patients and not just the most technologically advanced one.

REFERENCES

1. O'Donnell JK, Gladden RM, Seth P. Trends in deaths involving heroin and synthetic opioids excluding methadone, and law enforcement drug product reports, by census region - United States, 2006-2015. MMWR Morb Mortal Wkly Rep 2017;66(34):897–903.
2. Mack KA, Jones CM, Ballesteros MF. Illicit drug use, illicit drug use disorders, and drug overdose deaths in metropolitan and nonmetropolitan areas - United States. MMWR Surveill Summ 2017;66(19):1–12.
3. Daubresse M, Chang HY, Yu Y, et al. Ambulatory diagnosis and treatment of nonmalignant pain in the United States, 2000-2010. Med Care 2013;51(10): 870–8.
4. Florence CS, Zhou C, Luo F, et al. The economic burden of prescription opioid overdose, abuse, and dependence in the United States, 2013. Med Care 2016; 54(10):901–6.
5. The Council of Economic Advisers. The underestimated cost of the opioid crisis. Report to the President, 2017. Available at: https://www.whitehouse.gov/sites/whitehouse.gov/files/images/The%20Underestimated%20Cost%20of%20the%20Opioid%20Crisis.pdf. Accessed June 5, 2018.
6. Binswanger IA, Stern MF, Yamashita TE, et al. Clinical risk factors for death after release from prison in Washington state: a nested case-control study. Addiction 2016;111(3):499–510.
7. Binswanger IA, Blatchford PJ, Mueller SR, et al. Mortality after prison release: opioid overdose and other causes of death, risk factors, and time trends from 1999 to 2009. Ann Intern Med 2013;159(9):592–600.
8. Michna E, Jamison RN, Pham LD, et al. Urine toxicology screening among chronic pain patients on opioid therapy: frequency and predictability of abnormal findings. Clin J Pain 2007;23(2):173–9.

9. Couto JE, Romney MC, Leider HL, et al. High rates of inappropriate drug use in the chronic pain population. Popul Health Manag 2009;12(4):185–90.

10. Smith HS. Opioid metabolism. Mayo Clin Proc 2009;84(7):613–24.

11. Mortier KA, Maudens KE, Lambert WE, et al. Simultaneous, quantitative determination of opiates, amphetamines, cocaine and benzoylecgonine in oral fluid by liquid chromatography quadrupole-time-of-flight mass spectrometry. J Chromatogr B Analyt Technol Biomed Life Sci 2002;779(2):321–30.

12. Dams R, Murphy CM, Choo RE, et al. LC-atmospheric pressure chemical ionization-MS/MS analysis of multiple illicit drugs, methadone, and their metabolites in oral fluid following protein precipitation. Anal Chem 2003;75(4):798–804.

13. Wang WL, Darwin WD, Cone EJ. Simultaneous assay of cocaine, heroin and metabolites in hair, plasma, saliva and urine by gas chromatography-mass spectrometry. J Chromatogr B Biomed Appl 1994;660(2):279–90.

14. Presley L, Lehrer M, Seiter W, et al. High prevalence of 6-acetylmorphine in morphine-positive oral fluid specimens. Forensic Sci Int 2003;133(1–2):22–5.

15. Cone EJ, Clarke J, Tsanaclis L. Prevalence and disposition of drugs of abuse and opioid treatment drugs in oral fluid. J Anal Toxicol 2007;31(8):424–33.

16. Tennant F. Opioid serum concentrations in patients with chronic pain. J Palliat Med 2007;10(6):1253–5.

17. Tennant F. Opioid blood levels in high dose, chronic pain patients. Pract Pain Manag 2006;6(1):1–8.

18. Cone EJ, Dickerson S, Paul BD, et al. Forensic drug testing for opiates. IV. Analytical sensitivity, specificity, and accuracy of commercial urine opiate immunoassays. J Anal Toxicol 1992;16(2):72–8.

19. Bertholf RL, Johannsen LM, Reisfield GM. Sensitivity of an opiate immunoassay for detecting hydrocodone and hydromorphone in urine from a clinical population: analysis of subthreshold results. J Anal Toxicol 2015;39(1):24–8.

20. Fraser AD, Worth D. Experience with a urine opiate screening and confirmation cutoff of 2000 ng/mL. J Anal Toxicol 1999;23(6):549–51.

21. Osborne R, Joel S, Grebenik K, et al. The pharmacokinetics of morphine and morphine glucuronides in kidney failure. Clin Pharmacol Ther 1993; 54(2):158–67.

22. French D, Wu A, Lynch K. Hydrophilic interaction LC-MS/MS analysis of opioids in urine: significance of glucuronide metabolites. Bioanalysis 2011;3(23): 2603–12.

23. Dickerson JA, Laha TJ, Pagano MB, et al. Improved detection of opioid use in chronic pain patients through monitoring of opioid glucuronides in urine. J Anal Toxicol 2012;36(8):541–7.

24. Grabenauer M, Bynum ND, Moore KN, et al. Detection and quantification of codeine-6-glucuronide, hydromorphone-3-glucuronide, oxymorphone-3-glucuronide, morphine 3-glucuronide and morphine-6-glucuronide in human hair from opioid users by LC-MS-MS. J Anal Toxicol 2018;42(2):115–25.

25. Yang HS, Wu AH, Lynch KL. Development and validation of a Novel LC-MS/MS opioid confirmation assay: evaluation of beta-glucuronidase enzymes and sample cleanup methods. J Anal Toxicol 2016;40(5):323–9.

26. Feng S, ElSohly MA, Duckworth DT. Hydrolysis of conjugated metabolites of buprenorphine. I. The quantitative enzymatic hydrolysis of buprenorphine-3-beta-D-glucuronide in human urine. J Anal Toxicol 2001;25(7):589–93.

27. Elsohly MA, Gul W, Feng S, et al. Hydrolysis of conjugated metabolites of buprenorphine II. The quantitative enzymatic hydrolysis of norbuprenorphine-3-beta-D-glucuronide in human urine. J Anal Toxicol 2005;29(6):570–3.

28. Michael W, Dong KZ. Ultra-high-pressure liquid chromatography (UHPLC) in method development. Trends Anal Chem 2014;63:21–30.
29. Klepacki J, Davari B, Boulet M, et al. A High-throughput HPLC-MS/MS assay for the detection, quantification and simultaneous structural confirmation of 136 drugs and metabolites in human urine. Ther Drug Monit 2017;39(5):565–74.
30. Athar Masood M, Veenstra TD. LC-MS-sMRM method development and validation of different classes of pain panel drugs and analysis of clinical urine samples. Basic Clin Pharmacol Toxicol 2017. [Epub ahead of print].
31. Bodor GS. Quantitative, multidrug pain medication testing by liquid chromatography: tandem mass spectrometry (LC-MS/MS). Methods Mol Biol 2016;1383: 223–40.
32. Poklis JL, Wolf CE, Goldstein A, et al. Detection and quantification of tricyclic antidepressants and other psychoactive drugs in urine by HPLC/MS/MS for pain management compliance testing. J Clin Lab Anal 2012;26(4):286–94.
33. Mikel C, Almazan P, West R, et al. LC-MS/MS extends the range of drug analysis in pain patients. Ther Drug Monit 2009;31(6):746–8.
34. Krock K, Pesce A, Ritz D, et al. Lower cutoffs for LC-MS/MS urine drug testing indicates better patient compliance. Pain Physician 2017;20(7):E1107–13.
35. Fitzgerald RL, Griffin TL, Yun YM, et al. Dilute and shoot: analysis of drugs of abuse using selected reaction monitoring for quantification and full scan product ion spectra for identification. J Anal Toxicol 2012;36(2):106–11.
36. Dowling G, Regan L, Tierney J, et al. A hybrid liquid chromatography-mass spectrometry strategy in a forensic laboratory for opioid, cocaine and amphetamine classes in human urine using a hybrid linear ion trap-triple quadrupole mass spectrometer. J Chromatogr A 2010;1217(44):6857–66.
37. Marin SJ, Hughes JM, Lawlor BG, et al. Rapid screening for 67 drugs and metabolites in serum or plasma by accurate-mass LC-TOF-MS. J Anal Toxicol 2012; 36(7):477–86.
38. Depriest A, Heltsley R, Black DL, et al. Urine drug testing of chronic pain patients. III. Normetabolites as biomarkers of synthetic opioid use. J Anal Toxicol 2010; 34(8):444–9.
39. Fox EJ, Twigger S, Allen KR. Criteria for opiate identification using liquid chromatography linked to tandem mass spectrometry: problems in routine practice. Ann Clin Biochem 2009;46(Pt 1):50–7.
40. Varesio E, Le Blanc JC, Hopfgartner G. Real-time 2D separation by LC x differential ion mobility hyphenated to mass spectrometry. Anal Bioanal Chem 2012; 402(8):2555–64.
41. Dams R, Huestis MA, Lambert WE, et al. Matrix effect in bio-analysis of illicit drugs with LC-MS/MS: influence of ionization type, sample preparation, and biofluid. J Am Soc Mass Spectrom 2003;14(11):1290–4.
42. Chambers E, Wagrowski-Diehl DM, Lu Z, et al. Systematic and comprehensive strategy for reducing matrix effects in LC/MS/MS analyses. J Chromatogr B Analyt Technol Biomed Life Sci 2007;852(1–2):22–34.
43. Furey A, Moriarty M, Bane V, et al. Ion suppression; a critical review on causes, evaluation, prevention and applications. Talanta 2013;115:104–22.
44. Starrels JL, Fox AD, Kunins HV, et al. They don't know what they don't know: internal medicine residents' knowledge and confidence in urine drug test interpretation for patients with chronic pain. J Gen Intern Med 2012;27(11): 1521–7.
45. Reisfield GM, Bertholf R, Barkin RL, et al. Urine drug test interpretation: what do physicians know? J Opioid Manag 2007;3(2):80–6.

46. Reisfield GM, Sloan PA. Physician identification of opioid diversion: a difficult diagnosis. J Opioid Manag 2012;8(1):5–6.
47. Reisfield GM, Webb FJ, Bertholf RL, et al. Family physicians' proficiency in urine drug test interpretation. J Opioid Manag 2007;3(6):333–7.
48. Levy S, Harris SK, Sherritt L, et al. Drug testing of adolescents in ambulatory medicine: physician practices and knowledge. Arch Pediatr Adolesc Med 2006;160(2):146–50.

Matrix-Assisted Laser Desorption Time of Flight Mass Spectrometry

Donna M. Wolk, MHA, PhD, D(ABMM)[a],*, Andrew E. Clark, PhD[b]

KEYWORDS

- Mass spectrometry
- Matrix-assisted laser desorption time of flight mass spectrometry • MALDI-TOF
- Bacterial identification • Clinical microbiology

KEY POINTS

- Matrix-assisted laser desorption time of flight mass spectrometry (MALDI-TOF MS) is suitable for routine microbial identification in the clinical laboratory, and has quickly become an integral diagnostic tool.
- Rapid results provide microbial identification in support of antimicrobial stewardship programs, infection prevention, epidemiologic surveillance, sepsis campaigns, and other health care initiatives.
- Mechanics and processes underlying MALDI-TOF MS for microbial identification can be simplified for general laboratory understanding.

INTRODUCTION

Rapid and accurate identification of bacteria from clinical specimens is a critical function of the clinical microbiology laboratory. Historically, microbial identification depended on culture, biochemical testing, antigenic assays, or target-specific molecular for definitive identification. Matrix-assisted laser desorption time of flight mass spectrometry (MALDI-TOF MS), due to its high analytical sensitivity, is useful for microbial identification in the clinical laboratory. It exhibits high analytical sensitivity and has quickly become an integral diagnostic tool that drastically reduces the time required for definitive identification of bacteria, fungi, and mycobacteria from clinical specimens. Sample preparation is simple and reproducible, and results can be

Disclosure: The authors have nothing to disclose.
[a] Clinical Microbiology, Department of Laboratory Medicine, Diagnostic Medicine Institute, Geisinger Health, 100 North Academy Avenue, Danville, PA 17822-1930, USA; [b] Department of Veterinary Science and Microbiology, University of Arizona, Tucson, AZ 85721, USA
* Corresponding author. Clinical Microbiology, Diagnostic Medicine Institute, Department of Laboratory Medicine, Geisinger Health, 100 North Academy Avenue, Danville, PA 17822-1930.
E-mail address: dmwolk@geisinger.edu

Clin Lab Med 38 (2018) 471–486
https://doi.org/10.1016/j.cll.2018.05.008
0272-2712/18/© 2018 Elsevier Inc. All rights reserved.

labmed.theclinics.com

interfaced directly to the laboratory information system to provide rapid identification in support of antimicrobial stewardship programs, infection prevention, sepsis campaigns, and other health care initiatives. This article focuses on the technology and processes underlying MALDI-TOF MS for microbial identification and the associated downstream outcomes and improvements in health care related to its use.

HOW DOES MATRIX-ASSISTED LASER DESORPTION TIME OF FLIGHT MASS SPECTROMETRY WORK?

Background

MS has been used in the clinical laboratory for decades, but before the emergence of MALDI-TOF MS for microbial identification, its use had been largely relegated to high-complexity chemical analysis. The earliest attempts to use MS for the identification of bacteria occurred in the 1980s.[1] The MALDI ionization method was first introduced in 1987,[2] and was subsequently reported in similar experiments in 1988.[3] During the past decade, MALDI-TOF MS has become a rapid and highly reliable analytical tool for characterization of diverse microbes, such as bacteria, fungi, and viruses.[4–6] A variety of clinical and research-based laboratory methods and commercial instruments are available and are in widespread use across the globe; we describe the most common methods that are suitable for use in the routine clinical microbiology laboratory.

Sample Ionization in Matrix-Assisted Laser Desorption Time of Flight Mass Spectrometry

Microorganism identification by MALDI-TOF MS is dependent on ionization of proteins within the clinical specimen. MALDI is a type of "soft ionization" mechanism that uses transferred energy from a laser to generate protein ions for analysis. This mechanism is in direct contrast to so-called "hard ionization" techniques that transfer high levels of energy and can lead to fragmentation of the analyte. During MALDI, a chemically saturated solution of a low-mass organic compound (matrix) is added to the clinical sample (analyte). The analyte can be either intact bacterial or fungal cells, as in the case of intact cell MALDI-TOF MS (**Fig. 1**), or can be a protein extract from a designated clinical isolate. In some cases, direct blood culture broth, urine, cerebrospinal fluid, or protein extract are analyzed.[6]

Irrespective of the source, clinical samples are placed onto spots (ie, spotted) on a metal target plate and overlaid with matrix. On drying, the clinical sample and the matrix co-crystallize and form a solid deposit of sample embedded into the matrix. The plate holding the crystallized sample is then loaded into the MALDI-TOF instrument. The sample is exposed to a laser, present within a vacuum, which results in ionization of proteins in the sample (see **Fig. 1**).

The matrix is crucial for the successful ionization of the sample. The matrix acts both as a supplier of protons for ionization of the clinical sample, and as a scaffold, on which ionization can occur. Soft ionization of proteins is crucial when using MALDI-TOF MS for microbial identification, as it allows for the analysis of large biomolecules (ie, proteins) with sizes measuring up to 100 kDa without fragmentation.[2,3,7,8] The laser beam focuses on a small zone (usually 0.05–0.2 mm in diameter) on the metal target plate within the area where the sample/matrix mixture has been spotted and dried (see **Fig. 1**). An ultraviolet N_2 laser beam with a wavelength of 337 nm is used in most commercial MALDI-TOF MS instruments, including the Bruker microflex (Bruker Daltonics, Billerica, MA) and the Vitek MS (bioMérieux, Marcy-l'Étoile, France) (**Fig. 2**).

MALDI ionization is often found to be more sensitive than other ionization techniques. Irradiation occurs in short bursts of the laser to avoid damage or degradation

MALDI-TOF-MS
Sample Preparation

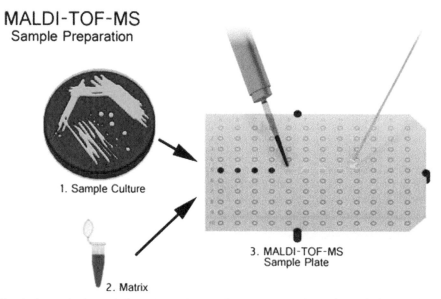

1. Sample Culture

2. Matrix

3. MALDI-TOF-MS
Sample Plate

Fig. 1. General schematic for MALDI-TOF sample preparation. (*Data from* Clark AE, Kaleta EJ, Arora A, et al. Matrix-assisted laser desorption ionization-time of flight mass spectrometry: a fundamental shift in the routine practice of clinical microbiology. Clin Microbiol Rev 2013;26(3):547–603. Copyright © American Society for Microbiology.)

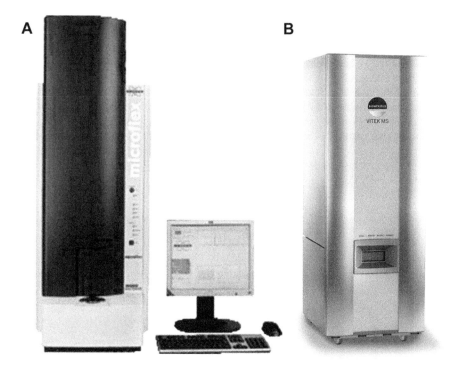

A

B

Fig. 2. Two common MALDI-TOF mass spectrometer instruments used in clinical microbiology laboratories (relative size, but not to scale). (*A*) Bexcton Dickinson/Bruker microflex instrument. (*B*) bioMérieux Vitek MS instrument. (*Courtesy of* [A] Bruker Corporation, and Becton Disckinson, Billerica, MA; with permission; and [B] bioMérieux, Marcy-l'Étoile, France; with permission.)

of the sample embedded in the matrix; longer exposures could cause rapid heating due to absorption of a large amount of energy from the beam causing heating and sample damage. The laser beam focuses on a small spot (usually 0.05–0.2 mm in diameter) on the metal target plate (see **Fig. 1**); therefore, adjusting the irradiance (ie, the intensity per unit of the analyte surface) is required and a beam attenuator is included in the laser optics of the MALDI-TOF MS instrument.

Analyte ionization is due to the uptake of energy from the laser beam, causing the dried matrix and clinical sample to sublimate (ie, pass from a solid phase into the gas phase, without passing through a liquid phase), forming a "plume" that contains ions from both the matrix and the clinical specimen (**Fig. 3**). Although the exact mechanism of ionization within the plume is unknown, it is best explained by a simplified 2-step mechanism consisting of primary and secondary ionization events.[6]

Matrices Used in Matrix-Assisted Laser Desorption Time of Flight Mass Spectrometry

Matrices used in MALDI-TOF MS are crystalline solids with low-vapor pressure that can easily become volatilized to form ions in a vacuum (as in the context of a mass spectrometer). The volume of chemical matrix exceeds the volume of the clinical sample, and that matrix to specimen ratio allows the production of intact gas-phase ions from large, nonvolatile, and thermally labile compounds, such as proteins. The matrix plays a key role in absorbing the laser light energy and causing a small part of the target substrate to vaporize. MALDI matrices should possess characteristics including (1) a strong absorbance at laser wavelengths used to facilitate ionization, (2) stability in a vacuum to force interaction with the co-ionized clinical specimen, (3) an ability to ionize the clinical specimen, (4) solubility in solvents that are compatible with clinical specimen, and (5) a complete lack of any chemical reactivity with the clinical specimen to avoid unwanted alteration or damage to peptides contained within the sample.

MALDI-TOF uses a UV laser, and the matrix molecule must incorporate a strong chromophore to help absorb energy and prevent protein fragmentation. Chromophores differ in their ability to absorb specific laser wavelengths; therefore, they are selected for use based on their ability to support electronic excitation of the matrix

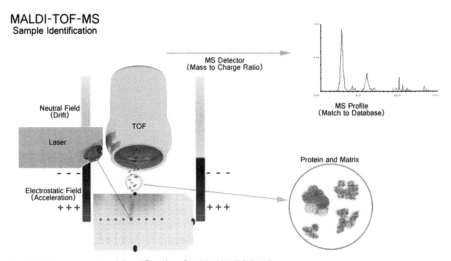

Fig. 3. Microorganism identification by MALDI-TOF MS.

in MALDI-TOF.[6] Commonly used for analyzing proteins and triacylglycerols, α-cyano-4-hydroxycinnamic acid (CCA), and its derivate 4-chloro-α-cyanocinnamic acid (Cl-CCA), are shown to be more efficient in proteomic analysis than other matrices[9] for clinical identification of infectious microorganisms.[7]

Time of Flight Mass Analyzers Characterize the Ionized Clinical Specimen

Following exposure to the laser, the ions generated from the irradiated matrix/clinical sample are analyzed, and their respective masses (ie, weights) and identities are determined. The mass analyzer functions to quantify and document the mass of the generated ions, supporting the identification of the proteins analyzed. The analysis reveals characteristic patterns representative of the clinical sample composition in the form of a spectrum of individual mass-to-charge ratios (m/z). m/z ratios are electrodynamic measurements of how quickly charged ions from the clinical sample move through the TOF tube and reach a detector, which in turn generates descriptive spectra of the ions that are detected (see MS profile, **Fig. 3**). The m/z ratios used for microbial identification are those from large ribosomal proteins that generate spectra that are unique to their respective bacterial species. Because these protein compositions among microbes are different, MALDI-TOF MS is capable of generating unique spectra for distinct species and (in some cases) subspecies. Comparison of the sample spectra to a curated spectral database leads to the identification of the microbe.

The TOF analysis is dependent on the principle of applying an electrostatic field (eV) to the ionized clinical material, which causes a generated ion with a charge (designated as z) to accelerate, imparting to it some amount of kinetic energy. The pulsed nature of the MALDI process pairs with the TOF mass analyzer, and all the generated ions enter the flight tube simultaneously.[10] The ions then move into a field-free drift region, where the only force affecting ion movement is the kinetic energy created in the acceleration step. The velocity of the ionized molecule from a clinical specimen can therefore be calculated. In the following equation, where m = mass, eV is the voltage applied, D is the distance to the detector, and t represents time, D and eV are constant, and t is measured, which allows the m/z ratio to be calculated[11,12]:

$$t = D\sqrt{\left(\frac{m}{2zeV}\right)}$$

This equation shows that the drift time is directly proportional to the m/z ratio. Larger ions will have a slower drift time, and smaller molecules will have a shorter drift time, demonstrating the separation of molecules based on mass.[13] This property allows for the separation of ions based on their corresponding m/z ratio. The MALDI-TOF MS method most commonly used in clinical microbiology laboratories is called linear TOF. In this method, the ions generated from the source accelerate into the flight tube, then enter a field-free region where they separate according to their velocities (and subsequently size), before hitting the detector (placed at the other end of the tube).

The Reflectron

A reflectron is a focusing element placed at the end of the TOF that changes the direction of ion travel. By applying a voltage to the reflectron's lenses, a change in the trajectory of the ions occurs, resulting in improved mass resolution. Ions with higher kinetic energy will penetrate the reflectron more deeply than those with lower kinetic energy. Therefore, the flight path of the high-energy ions elongates, which allows for averaging of flight times, and decreased peak broadening that is counterproductive to the process. Although a reflectron is effective at reducing peak broadening, it effectively doubles the ion path. For this reason, when analyzing high-mass ions with MALDI, a linear TOF is most commonly used rather than a TOF containing a reflectron.

MATRIX-ASSISTED LASER DESORPTION TIME OF FLIGHT MASS SPECTROMETRY USED IN CLINICAL MICROBIOLOGY LABORATORIES
Sample Preparation

Early studies evaluating the use of MALDI-TOF MS for microbial identification focused on the ability of the technology to accurately identify organisms to the genus and species level using whole microorganisms isolated from agar-based culture. Two different sample preparation approaches are used when performing MALDI-TOF MS: those that directly analyze the protein composition of microbes without sample processing, and those that use a protein extraction step before analysis. One of the greatest benefits of MALDI-TOF MS lies in the capability to eliminate labor-intensive protein extraction methods before analysis, allowing intact microorganisms to be directly spotted on a solid metal plate before analysis.[14,15] This process is known as intact cell mass spectrometry (ICMS).[15] Due to its simple sample preparation method, ICMS became an attractive alternative to phenotypic and molecular methods of microorganism identification.

By contrast, some microorganisms have more complex cell walls that can require additional manipulations before analysis. Ethanol-based inactivation, followed by preparative protein extraction using formic acid before MALDI-TOF MS analysis may aid in the analysis of some groups of organisms, including *Nocardia*, mycobacteria, and filamentous fungi. Furthermore, ethanol-mediated inactivation, or other methods to render microbes non-viable, is prudent from a biosafety perspective to prevent laboratory exposure to highly pathogenic microorganisms. In cases of suspected bioterrorism or select agents, inactivation via protein extraction always should be performed.

Spectral Databases and Software

The discriminatory power of MALDI-TOF MS is dependent on the content of the spectral database that the system queries to identify microbial colonies. Multiple spectral databases exist and manufacturers update and give support for their use. In some cases, databases can expand by populating the database with spectra generated within the local laboratory.

Vitek mass spectrometry software

The Vitek MS spectral database originated from the Spectral Archiving and Microbial Identification System (SARAMIS; AnagosTec, Zossen, Germany) database before being purchased by bioMérieux for incorporation into the Vitek MS platform in 2010. The database uses SuperSpectra assembled from strains from multiple well-characterized culture collections from diverse geographic locations. If no satisfactory match occurs using SuperSpectra, an expanded database with a broader collection of spectral information is queried to obtain a match to an organism already entered in the database. The software performs hierarchical analysis of the spectral data to determine relatedness of different microbial isolates to examine spectral changes within a population of related microorganisms, and to generate additional SuperSpectra for future database expansion.

Bruker Biotyper software

The MALDI Biotyper system was conceived and marketed by Bruker Daltonics and can analyze bacterial, mycobacterial, and fungal samples in addition to specimens recovered directly from positive blood culture bottles. Of all the mass spectral analysis software programs, the Biotyper platform is the most heavily used MALDI-TOF software package. The Biotyper software is an open platform allowing the user to save runs, construct Main Spectra (MSPs), and expand the database of stored spectra using tools included in the software. Mass spectra are analyzed for the presence of peak frequency, position, and intensity. Derived spectra are compared with a library of MSPs encoded in the Biotyper database. Like the SuperSpectra of the Vitek MS platform, these MSPs are derived again from replicative measurements of type strain with the goal of generating representative spectra of the organism across a range of biological variables. The user also can create Main Spectra with the aid of the software and populate the database with entries derived from microorganisms isolated in a local laboratory to better represent the distribution of microorganisms in different hospital settings.

ACCURACY FOR MICROBIAL IDENTIFICATION AND OTHER APPLICATIONS
Overall Performance for Identification of Common Microbes

Even under a condition in which culture medium or pH changes, MALDI-TOF MS is a highly accurate method for bacterial identification. Inter-laboratory comparisons are generally very good, as long as common and standardized reagents are used in the evaluations.[16–19] Most errors in published reports are thought to be the result of incomplete databases associated with the instruments, clerical error, or inability of the MS spectra to distinguish among similar species.[20–27] Widely accepted as a routine method for use in clinical laboratories, the accuracy of MALDI-TOF MS for identification of common microbes is undisputed and reviewed in recent publications.[6,28,29] We focus on emerging applications of this technology.

Performance for Identification of Mycobacteria Species

Beyond routine bacteriology and mycology, MALDI-TOF MS has become a useful tool for the identification of tuberculous and nontuberculous mycobacteria in clinical material. Technical refinements to sample processing have enhanced the discriminatory capabilities of the technology for mycobacterial identification, resulting in rapid robust identification of commonly encountered species using commercial systems.[30–32] MS peak analysis is also a useful tool for discriminating between closely related mycobacterial subspecies and members of species complexes.[33,34] Identification of mycobacteria by MALDI-TOF MS is also more rapid than hybridization and sequencing methods,[35] and is of value to laboratories that may not otherwise have timely access to such diagnostic technologies. Discriminatory power can be further enhanced through the construction of dedicated spectral databases or database expansion.

Direct from Specimen Testing

Although MALDI-TOF MS is considered a universal platform for identification of microorganisms isolated from culture media, the technology can analyze patient specimens directly, bypassing the need for culture and detecting the presence or absence of proteins from pathogens in the clinical specimen. Due to its highly sensitive nature, MALDI-TOF MS provides a method that can be used in place, of or in addition, to polymerase chain reaction–based methods for direct detection of pathogens from clinical samples. Both molecular and proteomic approaches to identify microbes directly are enhanced by preliminary processing to remove proteins, nucleic acids, cellular debris, and other elements that can inhibit analysis.

MALDI-TOF is a robust and accurate technology for the identification and characterization of single bacterial species present in direct urine specimens and has also been used, in a more limited fashion, to identify single bacteria in the cerebral spinal fluid.[30]

Direct identification of pathogens from blood culture broth is a promising goal with the potential to speed the identification process.[31,32] After preprocessing of blood culture broths to limit interference from blood cells and hemoglobin and to concentrate the microbes present, the procedure is like that of testing bacterial colonies. Identification by MALDI-TOF MS depends on the adequate concentration of the inoculum.[33–35] There is concern that mixed infections would be impossible to identify; therefore, Gram stain, in conjunction with MALDI-TOF MS is still necessary. Contrary to most protocols that try to identify blood culture broth as soon as the automated system detects growth,[25,32] some investigators have proposed storage of positive vials for 3 to 10 hours at room temperature if transport to a core laboratory site is required.[36] This strategy contradicts the urgency for identification of blood culture isolates.[37]

Early in its development, the lack of standardized protocols, use of different software for mass analysis, and different blood culture bottles made it difficult to compare the performance of different MALDI-TOF MS methods for direct identification. At first, the accuracy of the direct methods was shown to be 85% or less.[25,32,33,36,38–40] Later, as methods improved, accuracy for some species in blood cultures was reported to be higher than 85%.[34,36,41]

Vlek and colleagues[42] reported the implementation of MALDI-TOF MS in the laboratory has resulted in significant improvements to patient care when used for the analysis of positive blood cultures. In their trial, MALDI-TOF MS with the Bruker Biotyper software version 2.0 was used for blood culture broths, reducing the time to result by 28.8 hours and increasing the proportion of patients receiving targeted antimicrobials within 24 hours of sample collection by 11.3%.

Chen and colleagues[43] published the first study to compare 2 different MS platforms for the identification of microorganisms directly from positive blood cultures. They compared the Vitek MS (bioMérieux) system with the Bruker Biotyper version 3.0 for the identification of microorganisms from 202 positive BACTEC bottles. Sample processing, performed with the Bruker Sepsityper kit according to the manufacturer's instructions, allowed results from the MS system to be compared with identifications derived from 16S ribosomal DNA sequencing and phenotypic (Vitek-2) methods. The Biotyper system returned correct species-level identifications more often than the Vitek MS system and demonstrated better performance for gram-positive bacteria on the genus and species level. When analyzing polymicrobial specimens, both systems performed poorly.

For blood culture, the sample itself can pose difficult challenges when trying to identify the bacteria or yeast contained within. Components from human blood can cause interference or generation of noisy spectra generated by MALDI-TOF MS when analyzing direct blood culture specimens.[44] To address this issue, Bruker began standardization of sample extraction methodology by introducing the Sepsityper kit for direct analysis of bacteria from positive blood culture broths. In the first reported assessment of the Bruker Sepsityper kit, an analysis of 507 monomicrobial and polymicrobial blood cultures was performed to investigate the utility of the method. Gramnegative organisms were more accurately identified than gram-positive organisms, with significant difficulties reported for the identification of anaerobic bacteria, alpha-hemolytic streptococci, and polymicrobial mixtures.[45] Several comparative evaluations of in-house methods and the Sepsityper kit soon followed.[46–50]

Following initial description of the Sepsityper kit, Buchan and colleagues[51] sought to evaluate the performance of the kit in combination with MALDI-TOF MS for the identification of blood culture isolates using standard MS parameters. A total of 164 gram-positive, gram-negative, and fungal pathogen isolates were analyzed. The MALDI-TOF MS system with preanalytical preparation by the Sepsityper system identified 85.5% of isolates directly from blood culture. Results from gram-negative bacteria were more accurate than results from gram-positive bacteria, but genus and species concordance was comparable with the reference methods of Vitek 2 (bioMérieux) and Phoenix (Becton-Dickinson, Franklin Lakes, NJ) for both groups. Polymicrobial blood cultures and yeast identification remained a challenge. Adjusting the log(score) cutoff value to 1.5 improves identification of bacteria directly from blood culture.[49,52]

Fewer publications describe an attempt to standardize preparation methods for pathogenic yeast isolates recovered from blood culture,[53] yet the identification of bacteria and fungi directly from blood culture broth shows promise, potentially supporting for faster implementation of targeted therapy for patients with sepsis. For example, Lagacé-Wiens and colleagues[54] evaluated the Sepsityper system for the identification of bacteria from blood culture bottles and included an analysis of improvements in turnaround time and laboratory costs. Although limitations were reported for gram-positive and polymicrobial cultures, the mean reduction in time to report was estimated to be 26.5 hours. A comprehensive review of MALDI-TOF MS methods for the identification of microbes in the clinical laboratory is expertly reviewed elsewhere[55] and is outside the scope of this article.

Antimicrobial Resistance Testing

Although in early stages of development, several studies describe the successful use of MALDI-TOF MS for discriminating among antibiotic-resistant bacterial strains, improvements are being made to identify Enterobacteriaceae capable of producing extended-spectrum beta-lactamases,[56–59] carbapenem-resistant *Acinetobacter baumannii*,[60–62] carbapenem-resistant *Klebsiella* spp,[63,64] carbapenem-resistant *Bacteroides fragilis*,[65,66] methicillin-resistant *Staphylococcus aureus*, and vancomycin-intermediate *Staphylococcus aureus*.[67–71] and vancomycin-resistant *Enterococcus* spp.[72]

Strain Typing

Although rapid and accurate microbial identification by MALDI-TOF MS will attract laboratories to MS-based analysis methods, there is also the possibility for MALDI-TOF MS to provide epidemiologic data. One challenge faced by clinical laboratory scientists, infection prevention practitioners, clinicians, and public health laboratories is finding strain-specific data for the representative taxonomy of clinical isolates in outbreak situations.

Most strain-typing methods are complex and require a specialized laboratory infrastructure; therefore, these analyses are not routinely performed in every clinical laboratory, resulting in an increased quantity of "send-out" testing and delays in the investigation of hospital-associated infections and outbreaks. Sending samples to reference laboratories can result in delayed time to detection, loss of important epidemiologic data, increased testing costs, and potentially inaccurate or inconsistent results due to errors in specimen handling, processing, or transfer between laboratories. MALDI-TOF MS provides a mechanism by which much of the complexity in testing for minor changes in microbes is accomplished in near real-time. The use of

MALDI-TOF MS for strain typing is not routine, but as methods are modified to produce optimized, dedicated databases suited for the speciation and strain-level analysis of different microbes for epidemiologic and in-depth taxonomical analysis, the advantages that these types of data could provide to both hospital and public health officials is profound.

FUTURE VIEW AND IMPLICATIONS

Currently, some of the methods described here are still restricted to clinical research laboratories and large reference laboratories, but the potential of these testing algorithms to move into routine clinical microbiology and expand to include other microbial targets seems imminent, and impact is already being documented.[73–81] Implementation of MALDI-TOF MS into the routine clinical laboratory provides a powerful and accurate tool to quickly identify bacteria, mycobacteria, fungi, and *Nocardia* spp from culture. Further improvements in specimen processing of blood culture broths have occurred, and clinical trials have documented success.[78]

Laboratories face the challenges of implementation, selecting between MALDI-TOF methods and emerging molecular methods to identify bacteria from broth or direct specimens. Improvements to spectral databases and analysis software will further optimize the use of MALDI-TOF methods, perhaps reducing the turnaround time for identification of nearly all microbes. In the future, mass spectrometers will be linked with automated antimicrobial susceptibility systems, thus allowing for partial or complete automation of routine diagnoses. The first generation of automation resulted from collaboration with Becton-Dickinson.

In terms of speed and accuracy of microbial identification, integration of MALDI-TOF MS should change the current standards used in clinical microbiology laboratories. Optimal deployment of the methods could result in shorter hospital length of stay, improved clinical outcomes, and decreased associated health care costs. Rapid and accurate identification of microorganisms is becoming the standard of care, essential for optimal diagnosis and treatment of infections. MALDI-TOF MS technology may evolve to support direct testing but will require significant further research and method refinement. New clinical microbiology technologies are constantly changing to become a supplier of rapid, accurate, and actionable information, able to influence patient outcomes. As laboratories reduce time to results and improve accuracy and breadth of coverage, we extend the capabilities of these new methods. In partnership with basic scientists, novel technologies can evolve to help shape and define the diagnostic landscape for the future.

SUMMARY

Within the past decade, clinical microbiology laboratories experienced revolutionary changes in the way microorganisms are identified, moving away from slow, traditional microbial identification algorithms toward rapid molecular methods and MS. Historically, MS was a high-complexity method, adapted for protein-centered analysis of samples in chemistry and hematology laboratories. Today, MALDI-TOF MS, adapted for use in clinical microbiology laboratories, challenges current standards of microbial detection and identification. We are currently experiencing a moment in microbiological history when automated phenotypic and biochemical identification methods are surpassed by analysis of common proteins and genetic material. This article summarizes the capabilities of MALDI-TOF MS in diagnostic clinical microbiology laboratories and describes the underpinnings of the technology, highlighting topics such as sample preparation, spectral analysis, and accuracy. The use of MALDI-TOF MS in the clinical microbiology laboratory is growing, and, when properly deployed, can accelerate diagnosis and improve patient care.

REFERENCES

1. Anhalt JP, Fenselau C. Identification of bacteria using mass spectrometry. Anal Chem 1975;47(2):219–25.
2. Karas M, Bachmann D, Bahr U, et al. Matrix-assisted ultraviolet laser desorption of non-volatile compounds. Int J Mass Spectrom Ion Process 1987;78(0):53–68.
3. Tanaka K, Waki H, Ido Y, et al. Protein and polymer analyses up to m/z 100 000 by laser ionization time-of-flight mass spectrometry. Rapid Commun Mass Spectrom 1988;2(8):151–3.
4. Fenselau C, Demirev PA. Characterization of intact microorganisms by MALDI mass spectrometry. Mass Spectrom Rev 2001;20(4):157–71.
5. Lay JO. MALDI-TOF mass spectrometry of bacteria. Mass Spectrom Rev 2001; 20(4):172–94.
6. Clark AE, Kaleta EJ, Arora A, et al. Matrix-assisted laser desorption ionization-time of flight mass spectrometry: a fundamental shift in the routine practice of clinical microbiology. Clin Microbiol Rev 2013;26(3):547–603.
7. Albrethsen J. Reproducibility in protein profiling by MALDI-TOF mass spectrometry. Clin Chem 2007;53(5):852–8.
8. Hillenkamp F, Karas M. Mass spectrometry of peptides and proteins by matrix-assisted ultraviolet laser desorption/ionization. Methods Enzymol 1990;193: 280–95.
9. Jaskolla TW, Lehmann W-D, Karas M. 4-Chloro-α-cyanocinnamic acid is an advanced, rationally designed MALDI matrix. Proc Natl Acad Sci U S A 2008; 105(34):12200–5.
10. Cotter RJ. Laser mass spectrometry: an overview of techniques, instruments and applications. Anal Chim Acta 1987;195(0):45–59.
11. Vékey K. Internal energy effects in mass spectrometry. J Mass Spectrom 1996; 31(5):445–63.
12. Drahos L, Vékey K. MassKinetics: a theoretical model of mass spectra incorporating physical processes, reaction kinetics and mathematical descriptions. J Mass Spectrom 2001;36(3):237–63.
13. Cotter RJ. Time-of-flight mass spectrometry: instrumentation and applications in biological research. Washington (DC): American Chemical Society; 1997.
14. Holland RD, Wilkes JG, Rafii F, et al. Rapid identification of intact whole bacteria based on spectral patterns using matrix-assisted laser desorption/ionization with time-of-flight mass spectrometry. Rapid Commun Mass Spectrom 1996;10(10): 1227–32.
15. Claydon MA, Davey SN, Edwards-Jones V, et al. The rapid identification of intact microorganisms using mass spectrometry. Nat Biotechnol 1996;14(11):1584–6.
16. Mellmann A, Cloud J, Maier T, et al. Evaluation of matrix-assisted laser desorption ionization-time-of-flight mass spectrometry in comparison to 16S rRNA gene sequencing for species identification of nonfermenting bacteria. J Clin Microbiol 2008;46(6):1946–54.
17. Valentine N, Wunschel S, Wunschel D, et al. Effect of culture conditions on microorganism identification by matrix-assisted laser desorption ionization mass spectrometry #92. Appl Environ Microbiol 2005;71(1):58–64.
18. Wunschel DS, Hill EA, McLean JS, et al. Effects of varied pH, growth rate and temperature using controlled fermentation and batch culture on matrix-assisted

laser desorption/ionization whole cell protein fingerprints #93. J Microbiol Methods 2005;62(3):259–71.

19. Liu H, Du Z, Wang J, et al. Universal sample preparation method for characterization of bacteria by matrix-assisted laser desorption ionization-time of flight mass spectrometry. Appl Environ Microbiol 2007;73(6):1899–907.

20. Seng P, Drancourt M, Gouriet F, et al. Ongoing revolution in bacteriology: routine identification of bacteria by matrix-assisted laser desorption ionization time-of-flight mass spectrometry. Clin Infect Dis 2009;49(4):543–51.

21. Cherkaoui A, Hibbs J, Emonet S, et al. Comparison of two matrix-assisted laser desorption ionization-time of flight mass spectrometry methods with conventional phenotypic identification for routine identification of bacteria to the species level. J Clin Microbiol 2010;48(4):1169–75.

22. Mellmann A, Bimet F, Bizet C, et al. High interlaboratory reproducibility of matrix-assisted laser desorption ionization-time of flight mass spectrometry-based species identification of nonfermenting bacteria. J Clin Microbiol 2009;47(11): 3732–4.

23. Blondiaux N, Gaillot O, Courcol RJ. MALDI-TOF mass spectrometry to identify clinical bacterial isolates: evaluation in a teaching hospital in Lille. Pathol Biol (Paris) 2010;58(1):55–7 [in French].

24. van Veen SQ, Claas EC, Kuijper EJ. High-throughput identification of bacteria and yeast by matrix-assisted laser desorption ionization-time of flight mass spectrometry in conventional medical microbiology laboratories. J Clin Microbiol 2010; 48(3):900–7.

25. Prod'hom G, Bizzini A, Durussel C, et al. Matrix-assisted laser desorption ionization-time of flight mass spectrometry for direct bacterial identification from positive blood culture pellets. J Clin Microbiol 2010;48(4):1481–3.

26. Bessede E, Angla-Gre M, Delagarde Y, et al. Matrix-assisted laser-desorption/ionization biotyper: experience in the routine of a university hospital. Clin Microbiol Infect 2011;17(4):533–8.

27. Martiny D, Busson L, Wybo I, et al. Comparison of the microflex LT and Vitek(R) MS systems for the routine identification of bacteria by matrix-assisted laser desorption-ionization time-of-flight mass spectrometry. J Clin Microbiol 2012. https://doi.org/10.1128/JCM.05971-11.

28. Doern GV, Vautour R, Gaudet M, et al. Clinical impact of rapid in vitro susceptibility testing and bacterial identification. J Clin Microbiol 1994;32(7):1757–62.

29. Angeletti S. Matrix assisted laser desorption time of flight mass spectrometry (MALDI-TOF MS) in clinical microbiology. J Microbiol Methods 2017;138:20–9.

30. Nyvang Hartmeyer G, Kvistholm Jensen A, Böcher S, et al. Mass spectrometry: pneumococcal meningitis verified and Brucella species identified in less than half an hour. Scand J Infect Dis 2010;42(9):716–8.

31. La SB. Intact cell MALDI-TOF mass spectrometry-based approaches for the diagnosis of bloodstream infections. Expert Rev Mol Diagn 2011;11(3):287–98.

32. La SB, Raoult D. Direct identification of bacteria in positive blood culture bottles by matrix-assisted laser desorption ionisation time-of-flight mass spectrometry. PLoS One 2009;4(11):e8041.

33. Ferroni A, Suarez S, Beretti JL, et al. Real-time identification of bacteria and Candida species in positive blood culture broths by matrix-assisted laser desorption ionization-time of flight mass spectrometry. J Clin Microbiol 2010;48(5): 1542–8.

34. Christner M, Rohde H, Wolters M, et al. Rapid identification of bacteria from positive blood culture bottles by use of matrix-assisted laser desorption-ionization

time of flight mass spectrometry fingerprinting. J Clin Microbiol 2010;48(5): 1584–91.

35. Friedrichs C, Rodloff AC, Chhatwal GS, et al. Rapid identification of viridans streptococci by mass spectrometric discrimination. J Clin Microbiol 2007;45(8): 2392–7.

36. Stevenson LG, Drake SK, Murray PR. Rapid identification of bacteria in positive blood culture broths by matrix-assisted laser desorption ionization-time of flight mass spectrometry. J Clin Microbiol 2010;48(2):444–7.

37. Buehler SS, Madison B, Snyder SR, et al. Effectiveness of practices to increase timeliness of providing targeted therapy for inpatients with bloodstream infections: a laboratory medicine best practices systematic review and meta-analysis. Clin Microbiol Rev 2016;29(1):59–103.

38. Ferreira L, Sanchez-Juanes F, Munoz-Bellido JL, et al. Rapid method for direct identification of bacteria in urine and blood culture samples by matrix-assisted laser desorption ionization time-of-flight mass spectrometry: intact cell vs. extraction method. Clin Microbiol Infect 2011;17(7):1007–12.

39. Szabados F, Michels M, Kaase M, et al. The sensitivity of direct identification from positive BacT/ALERT (bioMerieux) blood culture bottles by matrix-assisted laser desorption ionization time-of-flight mass spectrometry is low. Clin Microbiol Infect 2011;17(2):192–5.

40. Marinach-Patrice C, Fekkar A, Atanasova R, et al. Rapid species diagnosis for invasive candidiasis using mass spectrometry. PLoS One 2010;5(1):e8862.

41. Spanu T, Posteraro B, Fiori B, et al. Direct MALDI-TOF mass spectrometry assay of blood culture broths for rapid identification of candida species causing bloodstream infections: an observational study in two large microbiology laboratories. J Clin Microbiol 2012;50(1):176–9.

42. Vlek ALM, Bonten MJM, Boel CHE. Direct matrix-assisted laser desorption ionization time-of-flight mass spectrometry improves appropriateness of antibiotic treatment of bacteremia. PLoS One 2012;7(3):e32589.

43. Chen JHK, Ho P-L, Kwan GSW, et al. Direct bacterial identification in positive blood cultures using two commercial MALDI-TOF mass spectrometry systems. J Clin Microbiol 2013. https://doi.org/10.1128/JCM.03259-12.

44. Stevenson LG, Drake SK, Shea YR, et al. Evaluation of matrix-assisted laser desorption ionization-time of flight mass spectrometry for identification of clinically important yeast species. J Clin Microbiol 2010;48(10):3482–6.

45. Kok J, Thomas LC, Olma T, et al. Identification of bacteria in blood culture broths using matrix-assisted laser desorption-ionization sepsityper™ and time of flight mass spectrometry. PLoS One 2011;6(8):e23285.

46. Juiz PM, Almela M, Melción C, et al. A comparative study of two different methods of sample preparation for positive blood cultures for the rapid identification of bacteria using MALDI-TOF MS. Eur J Clin Microbiol Infect Dis 2012; 31(7):1353–8.

47. Loonen AJM, Jansz AR, Stalpers J, et al. An evaluation of three processing methods and the effect of reduced culture times for faster direct identification of pathogens from BacT/ALERT blood cultures by MALDI-TOF MS. Eur J Clin Microbiol Infect Dis 2012;31(7):1575–83.

48. Martiny D, Dediste A, Vandenberg O. Comparison of an in-house method and the commercial Sepsityper™ kit for bacterial identification directly from positive blood culture broths by matrix-assisted laser desorption-ionisation time-of-flight mass spectrometry. Eur J Clin Microbiol Infect Dis 2012;31(9):2269–81.

49. Saffert RT, Cunningham SA, Mandrekar J, et al. Comparison of three preparatory methods for detection of bacteremia by MALDI-TOF mass spectrometry. Diagn Microbiol Infect Dis 2012;73(1):21–6.

50. Meex C, Neuville F, Descy J, et al. Direct identification of bacteria from BacT/ALERT anaerobic positive blood cultures by MALDI-TOF MS: MALDI Sepsityper kit versus an in-house saponin method for bacterial extraction. J Med Microbiol 2012;61(Pt 11):1511–6.

51. Buchan BW, Riebe KM, Ledeboer NA. Comparison of the MALDI biotyper system using sepsityper specimen processing to routine microbiological methods for identification of bacteria from positive blood culture bottles. J Clin Microbiol 2012;50(2):346–52.

52. Nonnemann B, Tvede M, Bjarnsholt T. Identification of pathogenic microorganisms directly from positive blood vials by matrix-assisted laser desorption/ionization time of flight mass spectrometry. APMIS 2013. https://doi.org/10.1111/apm.12050.

53. Yan Y, He Y, Maier T, et al. Improved identification of yeast species directly from positive blood culture media by combining sepsityper specimen processing and microflex analysis with the matrix-assisted laser desorption ionization biotyper system. J Clin Microbiol 2011;49(7):2528–32.

54. Lagacé-Wiens PR, Adam HJ, Karlowsky JA, et al. Identification of blood culture isolates directly from positive blood cultures using MALDI-TOF mass spectrometry and a commercial extraction system—analysis of performance, cost and turnaround time. J Clin Microbiol 2012. https://doi.org/10.1128/JCM.01479-12.

55. Hrabák J, Chudáčková E, Walková R. Matrix-assisted laser desorption ionization–time of flight (MALDI-TOF) mass spectrometry for detection of antibiotic resistance mechanisms: from research to routine diagnosis. Clin Microbiol Rev 2013;26(1):103–14.

56. Camara J, Hays F. Discrimination between wild-type and ampicillin-resistant *Escherichia coli* by matrix-assisted laser desorption/ionization time-of-flight mass spectrometry. Anal Bioanal Chem 2007;389(5):1633–8.

57. Sparbier K, Schubert S, Weller U, et al. Matrix-assisted laser desorption ionization–time of flight mass spectrometry-based functional assay for rapid detection of resistance against β-lactam antibiotics. J Clin Microbiol 2012;50(3):927–37.

58. Burckhardt I, Zimmermann S. Using matrix-assisted laser desorption ionization–time of flight mass spectrometry to detect carbapenem resistance within 1 to 2.5 hours. J Clin Microbiol 2011;49(9):3321–4.

59. Hrabák J, Walková R, Študentová V, et al. Carbapenemase activity detection by matrix-assisted laser desorption ionization-time of flight mass spectrometry. J Clin Microbiol 2011;49(9):3222–7.

60. Kempf M, Bakour S, Flaudrops C, et al. Rapid detection of carbapenem resistance in *Acinetobacter baumannii* using matrix-assisted laser desorption ionization-time of flight mass spectrometry. PLoS One 2012;7(2):e31676.

61. Hrabák J, Študentová V, Walková R, et al. Detection of NDM-1, VIM-1, KPC, OXA-48, and OXA-162 Carbapenemases by matrix-assisted laser desorption ionization–time of flight mass spectrometry. J Clin Microbiol 2012;50(7):2441–3.

62. Álvarez-Buylla A, Picazo JJ, Culebras E. Optimized method for *Acinetobacter* spp carbapenemase detection and identification by MALDI-TOF MS. J Clin Microbiol 2013. https://doi.org/10.1128/JCM.00181-13.

63. Tsai YK, Fung CP, Lin JC, et al. *Klebsiella pneumoniae* outer membrane porins OmpK35 and OmpK36 play roles in both antimicrobial resistance and virulence. Antimicrob Agents Chemother 2011;55(4):1485–93.
64. Cai JC, Hu YY, Zhang R, et al. Detection of OmpK36 porin loss in *Klebsiella* spp. by matrix-assisted laser desorption ionization–time of flight mass spectrometry. J Clin Microbiol 2012;50(6):2179–82.
65. Wybo I, De Bel A, Soetens O, et al. Differentiation of cfiA-Negative and cfiA-positive *Bacteroides fragilis* isolates by matrix-assisted laser desorption ionization–time of flight mass spectrometry. J Clin Microbiol 2011;49(5):1961–4.
66. Nagy E, Becker S, Soki J, et al. Differentiation of division I (cfiA-negative) and division II (cfiA-positive) *Bacteroides fragilis* strains by matrix-assisted laser desorption/ionization time-of-flight mass spectrometry. J Med Microbiol 2011; 60(Pt 11):1584–90.
67. Du Z, Yang R, Guo Z, et al. Identification of *Staphylococcus aureus* and determination of its methicillin resistance by matrix-assisted laser desorption/ionization time-of-flight mass spectrometry. Anal Chem 2002;74(21):5487–91.
68. Majcherczyk PA, McKenna T, Moreillon P, et al. The discriminatory power of MALDI-TOF mass spectrometry to differentiate between isogenic teicoplanin-susceptible and teicoplanin-resistant strains of methicillin-resistant *Staphylococcus aureus*. FEMS Microbiol Lett 2006;255(2):233–9.
69. Lu J-J, Tsai F-J, Ho C-M, et al. Peptide biomarker discovery for identification of methicillin-resistant and vancomycin-intermediate *Staphylococcus aureus* strains by MALDI-TOF. Anal Chem 2012;84(13):5685–92.
70. Wolters M, Rohde H, Maier T, et al. MALDI-TOF MS fingerprinting allows for discrimination of major methicillin-resistant *Staphylococcus aureus* lineages. Int J Med Microbiol 2011;301(1):64–8.
71. Josten M, Reif M, Szekat C, et al. Analysis of the MALDI-TOF mass spectrum of *Staphylococcus aureus* identifies mutations which allow differentiation of the main clonal lineages. J Clin Microbiol 2013. https://doi.org/10.1128/JCM.00518-13.
72. Griffin PM, Price GR, Schooneveldt JM, et al. Use of matrix-assisted laser desorption ionization–time of flight mass spectrometry to identify vancomycin-resistant enterococci and investigate the epidemiology of an outbreak. J Clin Microbiol 2012;50(9):2918–31.
73. Ge MC, Kuo AJ, Liu KL, et al. Routine identification of microorganisms by matrix-assisted laser desorption ionization time-of-flight mass spectrometry: success rate, economic analysis, and clinical outcome. J Microbiol Immunol Infect 2017;50(5):662–8.
74. Patel TS, Kaakeh R, Nagel JL, et al. Cost analysis of implementing matrix-assisted laser desorption ionization-time of flight mass spectrometry plus real-time antimicrobial stewardship intervention for bloodstream infections. J Clin Microbiol 2017;55(1):60–7.
75. Lin WH, Hwang JC, Tseng CC, et al. Matrix-assisted laser desorption ionization-time of flight mass spectrometry accelerates pathogen identification and may confer benefit in the outcome of peritoneal dialysis-related peritonitis. J Clin Microbiol 2016;54(5):1381–3.
76. French K, Evans J, Tanner H, et al. The clinical impact of rapid, direct MALDI-ToF identification of bacteria from positive blood cultures. PLoS One 2016;11(12): e0169332.
77. Mizrahi A, Amzalag J, Couzigou C, et al. Clinical impact of rapid bacterial identification by MALDI-TOF MS combined with the beta-LACTA test on early antibiotic adaptation by an antimicrobial stewardship team in bloodstream

infections. Infect Dis (Lond) 2018;1–10. https://doi.org/10.1080/23744235.2018.1458147.

78. Osthoff M, Gurtler N, Bassetti S, et al. Impact of MALDI-TOF-MS-based identification directly from positive blood cultures on patient management: a controlled clinical trial. Clin Microbiol Infect 2017;23(2):78–85.

79. Verroken A, Defourny L, le Polain de Waroux O, et al. Clinical impact of MALDI-TOF MS identification and rapid susceptibility testing on adequate antimicrobial treatment in sepsis with positive blood cultures. PLoS One 2016;11(5): e0156299.

80. Beraud G, Garcia M, Rahbari-Oskoui FF. Impact of MALDI-TOF will be highly dependent on the clinician. Clin Infect Dis 2013;57(10):1501–2.

81. de la Pedrosa EG, Gimeno C, Soriano A, et al. Studies of the cost effectiveness of MALDI-TOF and clinical impact. Enferm Infecc Microbiol Clin 2016;34(Suppl 2): 47–52 [in Spanish].

Proteoform Analysis to Fulfill Unmet Clinical Needs and Reach Global Standardization of Protein Measurands in Clinical Chemistry Proteomics

Yuri E.M. van der Burgt, PhD[a,b,*], Christa M. Cobbaert, PhD[a]

KEYWORDS

- Proteomics • Mass spectrometry • Clinical chemistry proteomics • Measurand
- Protein quantification • Proteoforms • Protein glycosylation

KEY POINTS

- Biomarkers play a crucial role in the pursuit of individualized patient treatment.
- Although genomic and transcriptomic analyses are of great value in the clinic, the complexity of the human body largely arises from variations in protein identities and quantities.
- Large-scale exploratory efforts have been applied on retrospective studies of (large) clinical cohorts of body fluids, such as plasma or serum samples, searching for novel biomarkers.

INTRODUCTION
Protein Biomarkers in Precision Medicine

In the pursuit of individualized patient treatment, biomarkers play a crucial role. Although genomic and transcriptomic analyses are of great value in the clinic, the complexity of the human body largely arises from variations in protein identities and quantities. In basic research, mass spectrometry (MS)–based proteomics has greatly contributed to an understanding of cellular functions at a molecular level.[1–3] Also,

[a] Department of Clinical Chemistry and Laboratory Medicine, Leiden University Medical Center (LUMC), PO Box 9600, Leiden 2300 RC, The Netherlands; [b] Center for Proteomics and Metabolomics, Leiden University Medical Center (LUMC), PO Box 9600, Leiden 2300 RC, The Netherlands
* Corresponding author. Department of Clinical Chemistry and Laboratory Medicine, Leiden University Medical Center (LUMC), PO Box 9600, Leiden 2300 RC, The Netherlands.
E-mail address: y.e.m.van_der_burgt@lumc.nl

Clin Lab Med 38 (2018) 487–497
https://doi.org/10.1016/j.cll.2018.05.001   labmed.theclinics.com
0272-2712/18/© 2018 Elsevier Inc. All rights reserved.

large-scale exploratory efforts have been applied on retrospective studies of (large) clinical cohorts of body fluids, such as plasma or serum samples, searching for novel biomarkers. Hitherto the number of new protein markers that made it from MS-based proteomics into the clinic is very limited.[4] Rather than having a technological origin, key reasons for this translation lag are the use of invalid samples, lack of thoughtful study designs, silo thinking of the stakeholders involved, and lack of appropriate test evaluation and adequate test standardization.[5] In clinical laboratories, proteins in body fluids are routinely tested for diagnostic and prognostic purposes as well as for therapy monitoring. It is, however, widely acknowledged that there is room for improvement with regard to sensitivity and specificity levels of current medical tests.[6] Moreover, clinically effective disease-specific tests that support diagnoses at an early and curable stage are still lacking for a wide variety of diseases. Aiming and searching for novel (protein) biomarkers should start by defining specific unmet clinical needs with the clinicians according to the test evaluation checklist.[5,7] Interestingly, post-translational modifications (PTMs) on proteins have often not been taken into account because of technical challenges and the increased complexity of the resulting data. PTMs on *existing* protein biomarkers provide an additional structural layer to quantitative levels of individual proteins with potential for patient stratification. Here, the often ignored presence of PTMs in protein tests and their implication for clinical chemistry proteomics (CCPs) are discussed.

What Is the Proteoform Hypothesis?

Comprehensive proteome information contributes to a systems-level understanding of human biology and, thus, disease.[3,8] Recently, interest in protein PTMs with regard to biological and clinical relevance has emerged as an additional layer in proteomics and has been coined as proteoform analysis.[9,10] The term *proteoform* was proposed in 2012 "to designate all of the different molecular forms in which the protein product of a single gene can be found"[11] and was swiftly adapted by the proteomics community. Although protein isoforms and PTMs are long known from gel electrophoresis and chromatography, in the early days of proteomics identifications (IDs) were based on so-called peptide (mass) fingerprints with the aim to determine *any* protein product from a single gene (and not *each*). An inherent effect was that the focus switched to the number of protein IDs and that isoforms were not considered anymore.[12] Since the beginning of this century, with the availability of the human genome, MS-based peptide sequencing has been optimized and turned into the method of choice for bottom-up proteomics (ie, identification of proteotypic peptides after digestion with a protease). Instrument development benefitted from the large growth in MS proteomics applications and was further developed with regard to speed and user friendliness. Moreover, these innovations led to ultrahigh-resolution platforms, such as orbitraps and Fourier ion cyclotron resonance mass spectrometers, that provide improved mass precision and accuracy and consequently yield more confident IDs.[13] Furthermore, these high-end platforms allow for a mass measurement of proteins in their intact form and offer a wide range of fragmentation techniques. So-called top-down proteomics studies have converged into a renewed interest in protein isoforms (ie, proteoforms) and have opened an exciting field within clinical MS.[10] Proteoforms arise from a single gene from changes due to genetic variations, alternatively spliced RNA transcripts, and PTMs (**Fig. 1**). An example of the last involves histone modifications that in a biological context are referred to as epiproteomic signatures.[14,15] Note that structurally related protein forms from different genes are not grouped together to ensure that the proteoform terminology remains compatible with a gene-centric approach.[16]

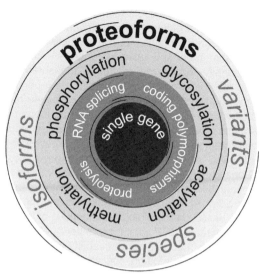

Fig. 1. Protein structural variants that originate from a single gene as a result of transcriptional processing and/or diverse posttranslational modifications. Proteoforms can, furthermore, arise from changes in the gene itself (allelic variants from coding polymorphisms or mutation). The terms *protein isoforms, variants,* and *species* are gray because these are ambiguous and do not accurately reflect the measurand of interest.

Soon after the first comprehensive proteoform analyses were performed and shown to be beneficial, the same group of Kelleher and colleagues[17] postulated a corresponding hypothesis, namely, that "intact proteoforms represent a powerful class of molecules for use as biomarkers of disease states."[17] Here the term *powerful* should be interpreted as "the ability to detect a true difference between two or more populations when such a difference is present."[17] The hypothesis refers to, for example, "detection of the presence or absence of cancers, the onset of disease, the classification of cell types or the differentiation of two or more biological states."[17] Indeed proteoform analysis provides a new layer of information that complements data related to transcription, translation, and posttranslational events that underlie complex phenotypes.[18] Genotyping and transcriptomic analysis are not telling the full story; for example, it was reported that mRNA abundances only weakly correlate with protein expression levels.[19] However, whether or not the proteoform hypothesis holds promise for clinical purposes partly depends on technological robustness and, moreover, has to be determined from measurements in large patient cohorts. In addition, methodologic challenges need to be overcome and requirements need to be met to show that proteoform-resolved data truly improve patient stratification.

Clinical Chemistry Proteomics and Metrological Traceability

Protein quantification in medical laboratories is mostly performed with commercially available, *Conformité Européenne* (ie, European conformity)–marked antibody-based immunoassays. For personalized patient care, accuracy of test results is essential; for correct interpretation, matching of reference values and/or decision limits is needed. In order to achieve standardized test results, metrological traceability is defined as "property of a measurement result whereby the result can be related to a reference through a documented unbroken chain of calibrations, each contributing to the measurement uncertainty."[20] Ultimate test standardization is reached when the entire reference system and metrological traceability chain are in place. This point is not trivial because the measured proteins often have a heterogeneous character (proteoforms). Moreover, commutable and value-assigned reference materials are often not available; internationally recognized reference measurement procedures are mostly lacking.[21] As a result, noncomparable results are reported between laboratories, for example, in the case of thyroglobulin.[4,22] MS-based technologies are the method of choice for tackling these issues, and recently steps toward harmonized MS-based measurements have been reported.[23–25] This approach is also used by working groups and committees of the International Federation of Clinical Chemistry (IFCC) for standardization of protein measurands (www.ifcc.org/ifcc-scientific-division/). Such MS-based targeted peptide measurements for protein biomarker quantification require analytical quality that is in agreement with their intended clinical use. A test that is fit-for-purpose should meet predefined analytical performance goals for bias and imprecision based on the biological variations of the analytes within and between individuals. Quantitative CCP aims for transfer of MS-based methodologies into a routine assay including metrological traceability with suitable calibrators and certified reference materials.[26] In addition, the aforementioned ultrahigh-resolution MS platforms allow detailed structural characterization of various proteoforms in the heterogeneous mixture of analytes, whereas in a medical test these may be interpreted as a single protein (ie, measurand). In an immunoassay *all* proteoforms that are recognized by the antibody, either biologically active or inactive, will be captured; as a result, a summarized protein quantity is obtained. Thus, in case the measurand is actually a mixture and is, therefore, undefined, standardization of immunoassays will be difficult to achieve. Proteoform analysis will not necessarily replace such immunoassays but certainly complement standardization efforts. Successful implementation of the traceability concept for quantitative MS-based CCP methods, along with unambiguous definitions of the measurand, should enable the development of traceable reference intervals and/or decision limits. Because of the heterogeneous character of the protein analyte in a medical test, the measurand can differ in the immunoassay and the CCP method; both require their own reference ranges and/or decision limits. With an increasing number of laboratories involved in quantitative MS-based CCP methods, external quality assessment and professional clinical chemistry organizations have started collaborations and joint projects to determine traceable reference intervals and/or decision limits for protein measurands.[27–30] In addition, these collaborations will deliver a template for further development of these MS-based methods into validated assays and finally clinical tests.

STRATEGIES FOR PROTEOFORM ANALYSIS
Proteoform Sampling, Separation, and Identification

An important aspect of any protein quantification experiment, but nevertheless often overlooked, involves the preanalysis part. Important considerations include specimen collection and transportation and sample handling and storage because proteins are not inert and sample degradation may be biased for certain proteoforms or yield new proteoforms (for example, due to oxidation or deamidation). With regard to sample preparation it is stressed that protein standards are often provided in buffer that is not compatible with MS analysis and that in these cases purifications may be needed to enable structural characterization studies. Obviously, an up-front proteoform separation simplifies sequential structure analysis; however, chromatography of intact proteins is more difficult than for any other biomolecule.[31] The first proteoform experiments were mostly based on offline purified proteins in which the mass analyzer was used as the separation device.[32] Such an approach remains valid; however, it is not attractive with regard to current high-throughput requirements, including well-defined reproducibility and robustness. Fortunately, progress has been made; nowadays online strategies have become available that provide proteoform separations. The two core technologies that are used involve liquid chromatography (LC) and capillary zone electrophoresis. Proteoform IDs are performed through bottom-up as well as top-down approaches.[33] The identification and quantification of proteins is routinely performed via MS-based bottom-up proteomics (also referred to as shotgun or peptide-centric) in which proteins are proteolytically cleaved (digested) into peptides that are most commonly separated by online LC and identified using tandem MS. With the development and introduction of quantitative CCP tests, the analytical specificity is enhanced; moreover, any clinically relevant proteoform can be detected and quantified. Essential elements for proper quantitative CCP standardization including metrological traceability are defining the measurands, selecting suitable proteotypic peptides, preparing labeled internal standards, optimizing proteolysis aiming for equimolarity between protein and peptide measurement, and calibration using well-defined internal standards and/or external calibrators. In top-down proteomics intact proteins are analyzed and characterized without digestion using ultrahigh-resolution MS platforms such as mentioned in the introduction of this article. Top-down MS provides information on the intact protein mass and allows for identification of novel proteoforms, in-depth sequence characterization, and quantitation of disease-associated PTMs. Top-down proteomics has given additional momentum for global and comprehensive analysis of proteoforms in existing (approved) protein markers as an additional layer of structural information.

Protein Glycosylation

One of the most common (and arguably complex) PTMs involves protein glycosylation. Most membrane and secreted proteins are known or predicted to be N- and O-glycosylated. Glycoproteins represent key molecules in many important biological processes, such as cell adhesion, endocytosis, receptor activation, signal transduction, molecular trafficking, and clearance, as well as in diseases, including cancer. In MS-based proteomics studies, this PTM has often not been considered for various reasons. First of all, whereas, for example, methyl-, phosphate- and acetyl-groups can be accommodated in database searches by an exactly defined mass difference, glycans are structurally diverse with different sizes (monomeric to oligomeric) and, moreover, can have isobaric identities. Consequently, glycan IDs require additional experiments, such as characterization of enzymatically released N-glycans or even orthogonal analytical strategies or instrumentation (eg, nuclear magnetic resonance spectroscopy). Secondly, to study the clinical relevance of protein glycosylation, the applied MS-based strategies require robust and high-throughput (HT) platforms that have only recently become available.[34] HT protein glycosylation studies are a type of proteoform analysis; consequently, this term is interchangeably used with the long-used glycoform.[35] In-depth approaches to determine site-specific protein glycosylation have become indispensable tools for functional analyses of these complex biomolecules. Protein glycosylation is known to change during disease and potentially offers a rich source of biomarkers. Discovery is either pursued on the level of a single protein by mapping all its proteoforms or by HT glycomics approaches. This first (single protein) approach is of interest for clinical chemistry purposes, because it can involve detailed characterization of an *existing* protein biomarker (as is pointed out earlier in the introduction section). A brief example is discussed in the applications section. With regard to the latter approach, the so-called total serum N-glycome (TSNG) comprises the N-glycans from all serum proteins, which are to a large extent liver- (acute-phase proteins) and plasma cell–derived (antibodies). Recent developments in MS-based HT glycosylation analysis have provided the opportunity to acquire information on TSNG N-glycan complexity, antennarity, galactosylation, and fucosylation as well as on the presence and linkage of sialic acids ($\alpha2,6$- vs $\alpha2,3$-linkage). Although these TSNG studies have yielded interesting glycan biomarker candidates for various diseases, exploratory efforts fall outside the scope of this article and are not further discussed.

APPLICATIONS IN CLINICAL CHEMISTRY PROTEOMICS

The benefits of clinical MS for protein quantitation have been pointed out and are increasingly acknowledged by clinical chemists.[27] As mentioned here, one of the major advantages involves test standardization according to International Organization for Standardization (ISO) 17511:2003, so that test results become traceable to standards of higher order and comparable among hospital laboratories. Test result comparability is essential in this era of electronic health records and free movement of patients across health institutions.[21,25] A second important driver for implementing MS-based assays in a medical laboratory is the ability to multiplex quantification of various proteins.[36,37] This ability is in line with current MS-based proteomics strategies that provide extensive lists of protein identities and quantities in clinical samples, such as tissue or body fluids. Here, the quest for a single biomarker in either retrospective or prospective study cohorts has turned into an approach in which protein signatures are aimed for or even full proteomes (ie, proteotypes) are reported.[38] However, the goal to fully describe a proteome is only partly met when listing large numbers of protein IDs. It has become clear that detailed structural knowledge on proteoforms has become a crucial aspect in many studies that involve proteome analysis.[39–41] The same holds true for the in-depth analysis of the heterogeneous character of protein measurands.

Multiple protein standardization efforts are carried out by the Scientific Division of the IFCC, wherein structural heterogeneity of the measurand needs consideration (see also the introduction). Although the biological and/or clinical importance of specific proteoforms has been demonstrated for certain proteins in the context of disease, it is also noted that validation of the clinical relevance of proteoform profiling requires further studies with larger patient cohorts. Examples of currently applied protein biomarkers that actually consist of a mixture of proteoforms are transferrin, apolipoproteins, and prostate-specific antigen (PSA). In the case of transferrin, it has been shown that abnormal transferrin glycosylation is known as a biochemical marker for the congenital disorders of glycosylation, a group of inherited metabolic disorders with defects in protein and lipid glycosylation.[42–44] Similarly, glycosylation profiling of transferrin is the cornerstone of the test for alcohol abuse (ie, carbohydrate-deficient transferrin).[45,46] In the case of apolipoproteins, these are constituents of lipoprotein particles and furthermore key-players in lipoprotein metabolism. Different glycoforms (ie, proteoforms) of apolipoproteins have an effect on lipid metabolism.[47,48] In the authors' laboratory, they have developed a quantitative CCP test for multiplexed measurement of apolipoproteins that has been applied in various studies on clinical cohorts for more than 3 years, such as on cardiovascular risk assessment.[49,50] It should be noted that in these quantitative CCP measurements of apolipoprotein C-III, all proteoforms with known as well as newly reported O-glycans (with fucosylation) are summarized into one value[51] (**Fig. 2**). It has been reported that sialylation levels of apolipoprotein C-III in serum associate with improved lipids for

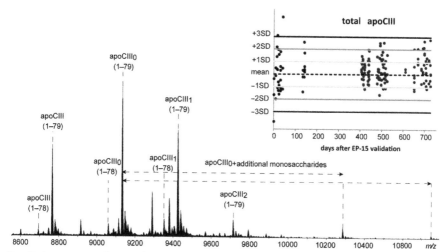

Fig. 2. Intact proteoforms of apolipoprotein C-III (apoCIII) in an ultrahigh-resolution matrix-assisted laser desorption/ionization mass spectrum (mass scale on the x-axis, 9 proteoforms are assigned). Proteoforms originate from protein O-glycosylation (subscripts 0, 1, and 2 indicate the number of sialic acids on the glycan; *monosaccharides* refer to fucosylation and glycan chain elongation) or from differences in protein size/length (numbers between parentheses reflect the amino acid sequence of apoCIII).[51] In the inset, a Levey-Jennings chart is shown of apoCIII quantities in a quality control sample measured over more than 700 days (on the x-axis).[50] On the y-axis, each value (determined via quantitative CCP) represents the sum of *all* proteoforms (ie, total apoCIII), whereas in the ultrahigh-resolution mass spectrum, each apoCIII proteotype is observed as a separate signal. EP, evaluation protocal; m/z, mass spectrometry; SD, standard deviation.

type 2 diabetes and prediabetes.[52] Proteoforms of apolipoproteins C-I and C-II have also been reported.[53] Such different proteoforms can potentially be included in the authors' laboratory-developed test.[37] The role of newly discovered apolipoprotein C-III fucosylation needs further investigation. As a side remark, the aforementioned quantitative CCP test also includes apolipoprotein E phenotyping derived from genetic variants within the patient cohorts. However, such phenotypes are not referred to as proteoforms because the variation is derived from differences in the genes.

A third example of a routinely applied protein biomarker that consists of proteoforms is PSA. Although the protein concentration of PSA in serum is an FDA-approved method for early detection of prostate cancer (PCa), its sensitivity is rather poor.[54] Currently, elevated PSA values (greater than 3 ng/mL or 4 ng/mL) are often followed by additional investigations, such as digital rectal examination, MRI, and/or prostate biopsy.[54,55] Moreover, the PSA test also lacks specificity because benign prostate hyperplasia or prostatitis can also result in elevated levels of PSA. Aiming for an improved PSA test, glycosylation of PSA has recently been described based on glycopeptide analysis, in which a total of 67 N-glycopeptides (proteoforms) were identified.[56] Here it was concluded that PSA proteoform profiling might be a promising tool for the determination of potential glycomic biomarkers for the differentiation between aggressive PCa, indolent PCa, and benign prostate hyperplasia in larger cohort studies.

FUTURE PERSPECTIVES

Proteins in body fluids are routinely tested in clinical laboratories for diagnostic, prognostic, disease classification, and monitoring purposes.[57] Yet, facing the large number of unmet clinical needs (eg, so far no tests are available for specific diseases like chronic obstructive pulmonary disease and acute kidney injury) and insufficient clinical performance of contemporary tests, there is room for improvement. MS-based methods in general, and quantitative CCP specifically, will complement total protein readouts obtained through immunoassays. In order to get this into place, a holistic and sustainable approach for demonstrating added value of quantitative CCP tests is needed, taking into account the concept of metrological traceability according to ISO 17511:2003.[21] The use of structured frameworks for test evaluation, such as the framework of the European Federation of Laboratory Medicine, guarantees that only tests that are *fit for clinical* purpose are developed and implemented.[5] Although some routinely measured proteins are successfully standardized at the global level, most protein tests are not yet standardized.[30] To this end, the authors pursue an integral approach to identify new protein markers as well as to measure existing markers by MS. In this context, it is stressed that biomarker translation and method transfer go hand in hand.

With this article, the authors aim to make laboratory researchers, clinicians, as well as in vitro diagnostic (IVD) manufacturers aware of the heterogeneous character of measurands in medical tests. To this end, knowledge of the identity and presence of various proteoforms in both reference samples and real-life patient samples is crucial both for a better understanding of the pathophysiology of disease for patient stratification and for enabling standardization according to the metrological traceability concept described in ISO 17511:2003. Proteoform analysis provides a stratification layer additional to quantitative levels of individual proteins or protein panels that already serve as biomarkers. The measurement of specific proteoforms may render MS-based strategies feasible as an add-on test to the corresponding protein quantification test. Proteoform profiling provides a golden opportunity for fulfilling unmet clinical needs in this era of precision medicine and for standardizing protein measurands at the molecular level in order to make test results comparable worldwide. Their analysis is of interest for the rapidly growing number of laboratory specialists and IVD manufacturers that acknowledge the potential of clinical MS and have shared their experience within the emerging community of MS applications in the clinical laboratory.

REFERENCES

1. Aebersold R, Mann M. Mass-spectrometric exploration of proteome structure and function. Nature 2016;537:347–55.
2. Altelaar AFM, Munoz J, Heck AJR. Next-generation proteomics: towards an integrative view of proteome dynamics. Nat Rev Genet 2013;14:35–48.
3. Hughes CS, Foehr S, Garfield DA, et al. Ultrasensitive proteome analysis using paramagnetic bead technology. Mol Syst Biol 2014;10:757.
4. Anderson L. Within sight of a rational pipeline for development of protein diagnostics. Clin Chem 2012;58:28–30.
5. Monaghan PJ, Lord SJ, St John A, et al, Test Evaluation Working Group of the European Federation of Clinical Chemistry and Laboratory Medicine. Biomarker development targeting unmet clinical needs. Clin Chim Acta 2016; 460:211–9.
6. Hoofnagle AN, Wener MH. The fundamental flaws of immunoassays and potential solutions using tandem mass spectrometry. J Immunol Methods 2009;347:3–11.
7. Horvath AR, Lord SJ, St John A, et al, Test Evaluation Working Group of the European Federation of Clinical Chemistry Laboratory Medicine. From biomarkers to

medical tests: the changing landscape of test evaluation. Clin Chim Acta 2014; 427:49–57.

8. Geyer PE, Kulak NA, Pichler G, et al. Plasma proteome profiling to assess human health and disease. Cell Syst 2016;2:185–95.

9. Smith LM, Kelleher NL. Consortium for top down proteomics: proteoform: a single term describing protein complexity. Nat Methods 2013;10:186–7.

10. Savaryn JP, Catherman AD, Thomas PM, et al. The emergence of top-down proteomics in clinical research. Genome Med 2013;5:53.

11. Kelleher N. A cell-based approach to the human proteome project. J Am Soc Mass Spectrom 2012;23:1617–24.

12. Nilsson T, Mann M, Aebersold R, et al. Mass spectrometry in high-throughput proteomics: ready for the big time. Nat Methods 2010;7:681–5.

13. Mann M, Kelleher NL. Precision proteomics: the case for high resolution and high mass accuracy. Proc Natl Acad Sci U S A 2008;105:18132–8.

14. Dai B, Rasmussen TP. Global epiproteomic signatures distinguish embryonic stem cells from differentiated cells. Stem Cells 2007;25:2567–74.

15. Young NL, DiMaggio PA, Plazas-Mayorca MD, et al. High throughput characterization of combinatorial histone codes. Mol Cell Proteomics 2009;8:2266–84.

16. The UniProt Consortium. Reorganizing the protein space at the universal protein resource (UniProt). Nucleic Acids Res 2012;40:D71–5.

17. Kelleher NL, Thomas PM, Ntai I, et al. Deep and quantitative top-down proteomics in clinical and translational research. Expert Rev Proteomics 2014;11: 649–51.

18. Aebersold R, Agar JN, Amster IJ, et al. How many human proteoforms are there? Nat Chem Biol 2018;14:206–14.

19. Khan Z, Ford MJ, Cusanovich DA, et al. Primate transcript and protein expression levels evolve under compensatory selection pressures. Science 2013;342: 1100–4.

20. JCGM200. International vocabulary of metrology – Basic and general concepts and associated terms. 2012. Available at: http://www.bipm.org/utils/common/documents/jcgm/JCGM_200_2012.pdf. Accessed at April 20, 2018.

21. Smit N, Van Den Broek I, Romijn FP, et al. Quality requirements for quantitative clinical chemistry proteomics. Translational Proteomics 2014;2:1–13.

22. Preissner CM, O'Kane DJ, Singh RJ, et al. Phantoms in the assay tube: heterophile antibody interferences in serum thyroglobulin assays. J Clin Endocrinol Metab 2003;88:3069–74.

23. Carr SA, Abbatiello SE, Ackermann BL, et al. Targeted peptide measurements in biology and medicine: best practices for mass spectrometry-based assay development using a fit-for-purpose approach. Mol Cell Proteomics 2014;13:907–17.

24. Annesley TM, Cooks RG, Herold DA, et al. Clinical mass spectrometry-achieving prominence in laboratory medicine. Clin Chem 2016;62:1–3.

25. Netzel BC, Grant RP, Hoofnagle AN, et al. First steps toward harmonization of LC-MS/MS thyroglobulin assays. Clin Chem 2016;62:297–9.

26. Lehmann S, Poinot P, Tiers L, et al. From "Clinical Proteomics" to "Clinical Chemistry Proteomics": considerations using quantitative mass-spectrometry as a model approach. Clin Chem Lab Med 2012;50:235–42.

27. Lehmann S, Brede C, Lescuyer P, et al. Clinical mass spectrometry proteomics (cMSP) for medical laboratory: what does the future hold? Clin Chim Acta 2016;(16):30246–7.

28. Sandberg S, Fraser CG, Horvath AR, et al. Defining analytical performance specifications: consensus statement from the 1st strategic conference of the European

federation of clinical chemistry and laboratory medicine. Clin Chem Lab Med 2015;53:833–5.

29. Dittrich J, Adam M, Maas H, et al. Targeted on-line SPE-LC-MS/MS assay for the quantitation of 12 apolipoproteins from human blood. Proteomics 2018;18(3–4). https://doi.org/10.1002/pmic.201700279.

30. Merlini G, Blirup-Jensen S, Johnson AM, et al, IFCC Committee on Plasma Proteins (C-PP). Standardizing plasma protein measurements worldwide: a challenging enterprise. Clin Chem Lab Med 2010;48:1567–75.

31. Chen B, Brown KA, Lin Z, et al. Top-down proteomics: ready for prime time? Anal Chem 2018;90:110–27.

32. Kelleher NL, Lin HY, Valaskovic GA, et al. Top down versus bottom up protein characterization by tandem high-resolution mass spectrometry. J Am Soc Mass Spectrom 1999;121:806–12.

33. Bogdanov B, Smith RD. Proteomics by FTICR mass spectrometry: top down and bottom up. Mass Spectrom Rev 2005;24:168–200.

34. Bladergroen MR, Derks RJ, Nicolardi S, et al. Standardized and automated solid-phase extraction procedures for high-throughput proteomics of body fluids. J Proteomics 2012;77:144–53.

35. Dell A, Morris HR. Glycoprotein structure determination by mass spectrometry. Science 2001;291:2351–6.

36. Van Den Broek I, Nouta J, Razavi M, et al. Quantification of serum apolipoproteins A-I and B-100 in clinical samples using an automated SISCAPA-MALDI-TOF-MS workflow. Methods 2015;81:74–85.

37. Van Den Broek I, Romijn FP, Nouta J, et al. Automated multiplex LCMS/MS assay for quantifying serum apolipoproteins A-I, B, C-I, C-II, C-III, and E with qualitative apolipoprotein E phenotyping. Clin Chem 2016;62:188–97.

38. Röst HL, Malmström L, Aebersold R. Reproducible quantitative proteotype data matrices for systems biology. Mol Biol Cell 2015;26:3926–31.

39. Nicolardi S, Bladergroen MR, Deelder AM, et al. SPE-MALDI profiling of serum peptides and proteins by ultrahigh resolution FTICR-MS. Chromatographia 2014. https://doi.org/10.1007/s10337-014-2812-8.

40. Trenchevska O, Nelson RW, Nedelkov D. Mass spectrometric immunoassays for discovery, screening and quantification of clinically relevant proteoforms. Bioanalysis 2016;8:1623–33.

41. Nedelkov D. Human proteoforms as new targets for clinical mass spectrometry protein tests. Expert Rev Proteomics 2017;14:691–9.

42. van Scherpenzeel M, Steenbergen G, Morava E, et al. High-resolution mass spectrometry glycoprofiling of intact transferrin for diagnosis and subtype identification in the congenital disorders of glycosylation. Transl Res 2015;166:639–49.

43. Marklova E, Albahri Z. Screening and diagnosis of congenital disorders of glycosylation. Clin Chim Acta 2007;385:6–20.

44. Hoshi K, Matsumoto Y, Ito H, et al. A unique glycan-isoform of transferrin in cerebrospinal fluid: a potential diagnostic marker for neurological diseases. Biochim Biophys Acta 2017;1861:2473–8.

45. Allen J, Litten R, Anton R, et al. Carbohydrate-deficient transferrin as a measure of immoderate drinking: remaining issues. Alcohol Clin Exp Res 1994;18:799–812.

46. Sillanaukee P, Olsson U. Improved diagnostic classification of alcohol abusers by combining carbohydrate-deficient transferrin and gamma-glutamyltransferase. Clin Chem 2001;47:681–5.

47. van den Boogert MAW, Rader DJ, Holleboom AG. New insights into the role of glycosylation in lipoprotein metabolism. Curr Opin Lipidol 2017;28:502–6.
48. Yen-Nicolaÿ S, Boursier C, Rio M, et al. MALDI-TOF MS applied to apoC-III glycoforms of patients with congenital disorders affecting O-glycosylation. Comparison with two-dimensional electrophoresis. Proteomics Clin Appl 2015;9:787–93.
49. Hermans MPJ, Bodde MC, Jukema JW, et al. Low levels of apolipoprotein-CII in normotriglyceridemic patients with very premature coronary artery disease: observations from the MISSION! intervention study. J Clin Lipidol 2017;11:1407–14.
50. Ruhaak LR, Smit NPM, Romijn FPHTM, et al. Robust and accurate 2-year performance of a quantitative mass spectrometry-based apolipoprotein test in a clinical chemistry laboratory. Clin Chem 2018;64:747–9.
51. Nicolardi S, van der Burgt YE, Dragan I, et al. Identification of new apolipoprotein-CIII glycoforms with ultrahigh resolution MALDI-FTICR mass spectrometry of human sera. J Proteome Res 2013;12:2260–8.
52. Koska J, Yassine H, Trenchevska O, et al. Disialylated apolipoprotein C-III proteoform is associated with improved lipids in prediabetes and type 2 diabetes. J Lipid Res 2016;57:894–905.
53. Trenchevska O, Schaab MR, Nelson RW, et al. Development of multiplex mass spectrometric immunoassay for detection and quantification of apolipoproteins C-I, C-II, C-III and their proteoforms. Methods 2015;81:86–92.
54. Wolf AM, Wender RC, Etzioni RB, et al, American Cancer Society Prostate Cancer Advisory Committee. American Cancer Society guideline for the early detection of prostate cancer: update 2010. CA Cancer J Clin 2010;60:70–98.
55. Mottet N, Bellmunt J, Bolla M, et al. EAU-ESTRO-SIOG guidelines on prostate cancer. part 1: screening, diagnosis, and local treatment with curative intent. Eur Urol 2017;71:618–29.
56. Kammeijer GSM, Nouta J, de la Rosette J, et al. An in-depth glycosylation assay for urinary prostate specific antigen. Anal Chem 2018. https://doi.org/10.1021/acs.analchem.7b04281.
57. Wright I, Van Eyk JE. A roadmap to successful clinical proteomics. Clin Chem 2017;63:245–7.

Harmonization of Liquid Chromatography–Tandem Mass Spectrometry Protein Assays

Alan L. Rockwood, PhD, DABCC[a],*, Mark S. Lowenthal, PhD[b],
Cory Bystrom, PhD[c]

KEYWORDS

- LC-MS/MS • Protein • Harmonization • Standardization

KEY POINTS

- Rigorous approaches to harmonization and standardization of clinical assays have been published.
- Less-formal approaches to standardization can serve a useful purpose of improving harmonization of liquid chromatography–tandem mass spectrometry (LC-MS/MS) assays before the completion of formal harmonization projects.
- Factors that can affect the harmonization process are discussed with particular emphasis on LC-MS/MS protein assays.

INTRODUCTION

Harmonization of diagnostic test results is fundamental to the effective use of laboratory testing in the diagnosis, treatment, and monitoring of disease. Working in an environment without any effort for diagnostic test harmonization might lead to diagnostic and therapeutic mistakes.

The International Consortium for Harmonization of Clinical Laboratory Results, convened in 2010, published a position statement[1] that defined 2 concepts; standardization ("uniformity of test results based on relation to a reference method") and harmonization ("uniformity of test results when a reference method is not available"). Although this statement is recent, it recognizes and elevates an old problem in

Disclosures: A.L. Rockwood and M.S. Lowenthal have no conflicts to disclose. C. Bystrom is an employee of Cleveland HeartLab.
[a] Rockwood Scientific Consulting, 11778 Stone Hollow Court, Salt Lake City, UT 84065, USA;
[b] Material Measurement Laboratory, Biomolecular Measurement Division, National Institute of Standards and Technology (NIST), 100 Bureau Drive, Stop 6315, Gaithersburg, MD 20899, USA;
[c] Research and Development, Cleveland HeartLab, 6701 Carnegie Avenue, Suite 500, Cleveland, OH 44103, USA
* Corresponding author.
E-mail address: alan@rockwood-scientific-consulting.com

Clin Lab Med 38 (2018) 499–513
https://doi.org/10.1016/j.cll.2018.05.004
0272-2712/18/© 2018 Elsevier Inc. All rights reserved.

laboratory medicine, the need for laboratory measurements to be equivalent within agreed and meaningful limits.

Several laboratory tests that have population-wide impact on human health have undergone this process (eg, cholesterol, glucose, hemoglobin A1c); however, few if any mass spectrometry–based methods have reached a level of harmonization or standardization presented in the American Association for Clinical Chemistry (AACC) position statement. In this respect, mass spectrometry (MS) is not unique because relatively few tests in the clinical laboratory have undergone the rigorous harmonization process advocated in this document. The present article discusses some of the issues relevant to MS-based assay harmonization and standardization with a focus on proteins.

APPROACHES TO HARMONIZATION AND STANDARDIZATION

Harmonization and standardization is a formal effort among a wide range of stakeholders that start with the definition of a clinically relevant measurand. Subsequently, measurement methods are obtained (or developed) and evaluated for their ability to reproducibly determine the measurand in patient samples. For methods that will ultimately be standardized, reference methods and materials are developed in parallel so that traceability can ultimately be achieved. A roadmap for this process has been described.[2] Key components of this approach are illustrated in **Figs. 1** and **2**.

Standardization takes the concept of harmonization to a higher level: methods are not just harmonized with each other, but also with an agreed-on absolute standard of

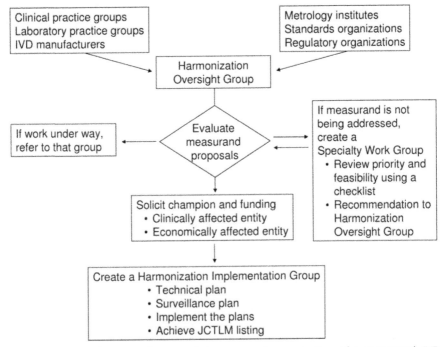

Fig. 1. Overview of a general approach to manage harmonization of a measurand. IVD, in vitro diagnostic; JCTLM, Joint Committee for Traceability of Laboratory Medicine. Greg Miller W, Myers GL, Lou Gantzer M, et al. Roadmap for Harmonization of Clinical Laboratory Measurement Procedures Clinical Chemistry 2011;57(8):1108–17; *Reproduced with permission from* the American Association for Clinical Chemistry.

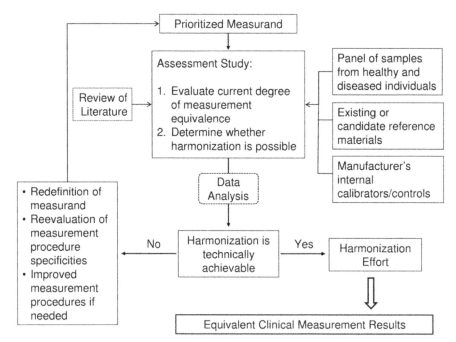

Fig. 2. General process for assessing and achieving harmonization (equivalency) of clinical laboratory measurement results. Greg Miller W, Myers GL, Lou Gantzer M, et al. Roadmap for Harmonization of Clinical Laboratory Measurement Procedures Clinical Chemistry 2011;57(8):1108–17; *Reproduced with permission from* the American Association for Clinical Chemistry.

accuracy. Based on concepts outlined in ISO 17511:2003, a fully standardized method includes a traceability chain that is often presented in the form of a diagram mapping out a hierarchy of materials and procedures providing traceability of results back to a primary standard (**Fig. 3**).

The top of the traceability chain begins with definition of SI units for a selected measurand. On the left-hand side of the ladder we have derived materials used for measurement, while on the right-hand side we have a series of measurement methods. At each step of the ladder from top to bottom, materials and methods are fully evaluated so that trueness and imprecision can be accounted for. From a practical point of view, routine laboratory measurements at the bottom of the hierarchy are typically performed in high volumes and with the largest uncertainty, but under this scheme the measurement can be ensured not to exceed an established error budget.

The schemes summarized in **Figs. 1–3** represent an aspirational goal for fully harmonized and/or standardized methods, although relatively few methods in clinical chemistry have completed this rigorous process to date, and to our knowledge no routine MS-based methods are among these fully harmonized or standardized methods, although in the small-molecule realm, significant progress toward that goal has been made by laboratories that have voluntarily participated in the Centers for disease Control and Prevention's (CDC's) Hormone Standardization (HoSt) Program[3] and Vitamin D Standardization-Certification Program (VDSCP).[4]

Although the roadmap provides a starting point for planning a formal harmonization project, it makes evident that this is a large-scale project best suited to commercially produced assays from multiple vendors, and such efforts may take many years or

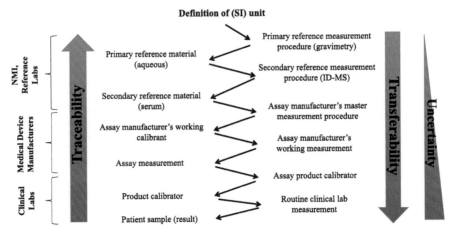

Fig. 3. Illustration of traceability chain for standardizing methods to an agreed-on absolute standard of accuracy. NMI, National Measurement Institute. (*Data from* International Organization for Standardization. (2003–2008). In vitro diagnostic medical devices – Measurement of quantities in biological samples – Metrological traceability of values assigned to calibrators and control materials (ISO 17511:2003). Retrieved from: https://www.iso.org/standard/30716.html)

even decades to bear fruit, but more informal harmonization investigations carried out in laboratories before full-scale harmonization or standardization efforts also have value.

DEFINING THE MEASURAND

Seldom, if ever, does a protein exist in a single form. Rather numerous proteoforms encompass protein variability that arise in the process of transcription, translation, and posttranslational modification. For harmonization efforts to be clinically relevant, it is essential that the appropriate proteoform(s) be targeted by the analytical method. Defining the appropriate measurand requires extensive research and can impact harmonization of liquid chromatography–tandem MS (LC-MS/MS) methods in multiple ways, some favorable and some unfavorable.

MS-based detection is highly capable of differentiating heterogeneous proteoforms. These methods may be general, targeting a wide variety of proteoforms, or more narrowly targeted on a subset of proteoforms. Regardless of which proteoforms are selected, they should be relevant to the clinical needs.

Brain natriuretic peptide (BNP) is a good example. It is secreted as a 108-amino acid prohormone (proBNP) and is useful as a biomarker to rule out acute heart failure in an emergency setting. However, harmonization of current immunoassay platforms for BNP are problematic due to variability of cross-reactivity for different forms of BNP for assays from different vendors. The variable analytical specificity of immunoassay platforms is one limiting factor to establishing harmonized BNP results.[5] MS approaches may be more capable of addressing the complex metabolism of the natriuretic peptide family, and identify diagnostically relevant forms.

REAGENTS FOR HARMONIZATION

A foundation for harmonization is agreement on an appropriate material against which test methods can be compared. From a bioanalytical perspective, the ideal material is a fully characterized pure protein, biochemically and biophysically identical to the native protein, which retains these same properties when added to a realistic matrix in required proportions. This ideal situation would allow for highly accurate and reproducible manufacture of reference material.

Achieving this goal is exceptionally challenging. Reference material manufactured using recombinant protein can have limitations, often lacking natural posttranslational modifications (phosphorylation, glycosylation), and recombinant proteins may lack the correct tertiary or quaternary structure.

As an alternative approach, purified native proteins and/or native matrix can arguably have better agreement in terms of biochemical and structural features, but biological variability arising from donor pool differences and matrix-dependent challenges in purification can result in unwanted lot-to-lot variability. Fully native matrix also presents challenges in how to achieve controlled differences in levels if required.

In practice, there are 2 broad types of materials used for harmonization of protein assays: recombined materials prepared with highly purified naturally occurring or recombinant protein added to measurand-free matrix, or fully native matrix in which the measurand has been highly characterized. The National Institute for Biological Standards and Control (NIBSC), European Joint Research Center (JRC), National Institute of Standards and Technology (NIST), National Metrology Institute of Japan, and others provide certified standards and reference materials for a wide range of clinically important protein and peptide analytes (eg, IGF-1, NIBSC code 02/254; Insulin, NIBSC code 83/500; ApoA-I, JRC BCR-393; C-reactive protein, NIST SRM 2924; cTnI, NIST SRM 2921).

In any case, 2 challenges that must always be addressed when harmonizing against a reference material are how to assign a value to the reference material and how to ensure commutability of the reference material. These issues must be addressed when setting up and executing a harmonization project.

MASS SPECTROMETRY AS A PREFERRED PLATFORM FOR HARMONIZATION AND STANDARDIZATION

MS is a platform especially well-suited for assay harmonization, both with regard to reference methods within a standardization program and as routine methods used for routine analysis of patient samples. First, although multiple vendors supply the market with a range of instruments with varying performance, each system operates from the same first principles. The physics of generating, focusing, filtering, and transmitting ions for detection use similar principles across vendors, which affords much similarity between instruments. This contrasts with other common technologies, in which detection and instrument systems can vary dramatically for the same analyte (eg, turbidometry, spectrophotometry, fluorometry, electrochemiluminescence, and chemiluminescence).

Second, MS relies on direct detection of specific molecules or molecular fragments based on a well-defined and easily understood physical property, that is, mass. In this case, the identity of the species used for detection and quantification can be determined using well-established principles and procedures, such as interpretation of tandem mass spectra and accurate mass measurements, either by de novo methods or by comparison against known standards. By way of contrast, detection in immunometric systems relies on the recognition of an epitope by an antibody, which is at heart a problem in natural product chemistry and is therefore subject to much uncertainty. Despite the ability to produce antibodies with high avidity and selectivity, the tremendous complexity of a matrix like human serum, as well as the relative irreproducibility of antibody production and characterization, makes guarantee of consistent fidelity challenging. Finally, the ability to incorporate heavy isotopes to prepare labeled internal standards substantially improves assay accuracy and precision in MS as well as providing insight into assay performance and quality control, which is difficult to replicate using other measurement techniques.

The combination of these advantages is often applied to the development of reference methods using isotope dilution (ID) techniques with LC-MS/MS. A common approach for harmonizing assays is to quantify protein measurands through a "bottom-up" workflow by detection of surrogate peptides that result from a proteolytic digestion of the clinically relevant protein. ID requires the use of heavy-isotope–labeled internal standards spiked into biological samples and into calibration standards, facilitating high-precision, low-bias quantification. Multiple-reaction monitoring (MRM) MS using a triple-quadrupole instrument is a highly selective technique that allows simultaneous, multiplexed detection of natural and heavy (ie, labeled) forms of surrogate peptides detected by precursor-to-fragment ion transitions. Whereas synthetic labeled peptides are appropriate for use in some applications, other harmonization efforts will require full-length recombinantly produced protein internal standards, a manufacturing challenge in itself.

The general strategy for protein quantification meant to underpin harmonization efforts has been established for LC-MS techniques. Yet to date, only a few reference measurement methods (RMs) for proteins have been developed using ID LC-MS/MS techniques. These internationally accepted RMs include clinical markers, such as amyloid beta 1 to 42, HbA1c, and C-peptide. As MS has become more widely available, the possibility of deploying routine methods with analytical performance close to that expected from reference methods has become possible. Despite the analytical utility of MS, development of methods with exemplary performance requires extensive knowledge, extensive development, and exhaustive validation.

COMMUTABILITY AND MATRIX EFFECTS

A key requirement in any standardization program is that the reference materials must be analytically equivalent to the target compounds in patient samples, or in other words, commutability is a key issue, and matrix effects must be minimal or absent. We often think of poor commutability as primarily affecting immunoassays, but one must not overlook the fact that it can also affect MS-based assays. To illustrate this with 2 examples, electrospray ionization, which is widely used in the clinical laboratory, is subject to matrix-dependent suppression of ionization efficiency. To a large extent, the use of internal standards can overcome this issue, but if ion suppression is too severe, the signal levels may become too low to be usable. As a second example, it has become generally accepted that one should use ratios of ion abundances from different MS/MS transitions to detect the presence of interferences. Briefly, when this ratio for a patient sample differs from that of a pure standard, an interfering compound is deemed likely. However, experiments have shown cases in which the branching ratios for different MS/MS pathways can be matrix dependent.[6,7] In any standardization program, even those targeted to MS-based methods, the materials and methods must be rigorously evaluated for commutability and matrix effects.[8–10]

EXAMPLES

This section discusses examples of both preliminary informal harmonization efforts and more formal harmonization efforts. Thyroglobulin (Tg) and insulin-like growth factor-1 (IGF-1) both represent important clinical markers that attracted interest in de novo test development by LC-MS/MS. Tg is a marker for thyroid cancer recurrence. After thyroidectomy, circulating levels of Tg are expected to decline to undetectable levels unless there is recurrence of disease. A recognized limitation of the immunometric measurement of Tg is the high proportion of patients who have circulating autoantibodies directed against Tg.

Measurement of IGF-1 is used in the diagnosis of growth disorders. This protein measurand circulates as a complex with IGF binding proteins. Much like autoantibodies, the presence of binding proteins makes accurate and precise quantification of IGF-1 by immunoassay difficult.

First let us consider Tg as a model for an informal preliminary approach to harmonization. It should be noted at the outset that the Tg work referenced here[11,12] was essentially a method comparison study presented as a first step toward harmonization, and not as a full harmonization project, either formal or informal. For example, that study did not include the process of selecting an agreed-on reference material or reference method. Furthermore, we recognize that reasonable people may disagree on whether informal/preliminary harmonization efforts should be pursued at all.

Within the past decade, methods for Tg analysis by LC-MS/MS were under independent development by several laboratories. Within a relatively short time, several laboratories introduced their versions of Tg analysis by LC-MS/MS. Although similar in certain broad features (each using a surrogate peptide from a tryptic digest, for example), the method details varied substantially. To provide the best patient care possible, several of these laboratories, which were otherwise strongly competitive with each other, agreed to participate in a multi-laboratory method comparison study and to publish the results.

Fig. 4 summarizes the results from these studies. Necessarily, each laboratory had to initially pick some method or reference material to which to anchor their results.

The graph on the left presents the results for 4 LC-MS/MS methods compared with the average of the 4 methods. The graph on the right compares 4 well-established immunoassays. It is immediately obvious that the LC-MS/MS methods compare with each other at least as well as the immunoassays compare with each other, and probably better. Of particular relevance, compared with the immunoassays-based methods, the LC-MS/MS methods showed better agreement with each other when

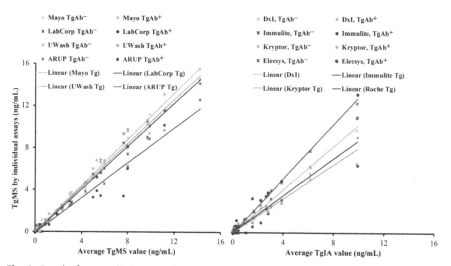

Fig. 4. Results from preliminary Tg harmonization study. (*From* Netzel BC, Grant RP, Hoofnagle AN. First steps toward harmonization of LC-MS/MS thyroglobulin assays: letter to the editor. Clin Chem 2015;62:1; with permission.)

autoantibodies were present, which was the primary motivation for developing the LC-MS/MS methods to begin with. The agreement among the 4 LC-MS/MS methods is remarkable considering the detailed differences between the LC-MS/MS procedures described in the article.

In a similar vein, measurement of IGF-1 was evaluated among 4 international laboratories that independently developed LC-MS/MS methods and subsequently examined the consequences of various calibration strategies, which included the use of an NIBSC reference material. Similar to the findings for Tg, careful de novo assay development yielded intra-laboratory agreement that was better than observed using a commercial platform in 2 different laboratories.

One can take important lessons from these 2 examples. First, even though there were no established LC-MS/MS-based methods for comparison when the assays were under development, the potential for good harmonization was baked into them via choice of calibrators, as described in the article, as well as certain advantages inherent in MS-based methods, as discussed in the present article.

A second lesson from Tg is that given that these 4 assays were all being offered for patient care, it was important not to wait for a larger-scale harmonization program to be implemented before beginning some kind of harmonization effort. Part of the background to this is that the MS-based methods were developed to improve patient care (ie, deal with the problem of interference by autoantibodies in immunoassays), and in light of this it seemed inappropriate to wait years for a large-scale harmonization project before putting these assays into service.

Third, the study investigators explicitly recognized that this was a preliminary effort and that higher-level harmonization studies should be done.

Fourth, even though these laboratories operate in a competitive environment, all recognized the importance of working together in this area to provide the best patient care possible.

The approach used for the preliminary Tg harmonization can serve a model for other LC-MS/MS methods of protein analysis. Elements of this approach, some of which were foreshadowed in the last paragraph, include the following: (1) Although all laboratories may have a hand in structuring the study, it is important to have 1 person at 1 institution assigned to lead the process and to keep the process on track. (2) The classifications of samples used in the study should address potential issues or potential weaknesses relevant to a method. For example, the Tg study included a group of samples for which autoantibodies against Tg were present. This issue had already been identified as a possible weakness for immunoassays, and given that the MS-based method purported to overcome interferences arising from autoantibodies, it was important to address this issue in a harmonization study over multiple laboratories. (3) Performance parameters to be compared must be agreed on. Obviously, this would normally include comparison of quantitative results, but depending on the situation may include other parameters, such lower limits of quantification. In the case of the Tg study, the lower limits of quantification were not compared, although the laboratories were transparent with regard to that specification. (4) The study members must agree to the number of samples to be used, what will be the sources of the samples, and the procedures used to share the samples. (5) In many cases, laboratory competition is an underlying issue that needs to be dealt with. Ideally, all laboratories offering a particular protein LC-MS/MS assay will agree to be involved in the study. In the case of Tg, most but not all of the laboratories offering the test at that time participated in the study. Furthermore, in the interest of transparency, the participating laboratories agreed to participate in the study nonanonymously and to have the results published in the open literature. Relevant to the competitiveness, intellectual property issues may sometimes make cooperation difficult, but for the good of the patient, it is important to try to work these issues out. (6) The participants should be aware that an early-phase method comparison is just a step toward the ultimate goal of a high-level harmonization program, or in the best case, a full standardization program, while at the same time recognizing that these higher-level harmonization goals may be years away.

A recent publication[13] illustrates a more formalized example of approaches to harmonization. This article is highly recommended for its discussion of formal harmonization processes applied to the real-life example of C-peptide. Among other things, that article provides a historical narrative of efforts to standardize C-peptide, starting in 2002 with the formation of a C-peptide Standardization Committee by the National Institute of Diabetes and Digestive and Kidney Diseases in the United States. The Diabetes Diagnostic Laboratory at the University of Missouri coordinated the effort that eventually became an international effort involving multiple agencies. The study was not focused specifically on standardization of MS-based end-user methods for C-peptide, but would apply to all methods for C-peptide. However, that work did eventually lead to an MS-based reference method for C-peptide. The development of a reference method has been an essential part of the harmonization program, but in-and-of-itself does not complete the process of assay standardization, and the article lays out some steps to be taken in the future specific to the reference method itself.

This article draws several lessons, starting with the fact that someone has to pay for the work. Also noted is that communication among the many groups involved in the effort can be difficult. Other lessons are that the goals should be laid out at the beginning of the process, that the time frame for successful formal harmonization is long (more than a decade and a half so far in this example, and the standardization process is yet to be completed), and that the development of reference materials and procedures can be long, difficult, and expensive. The most fundamental lesson was left unstated in the article, which is that the process started with the fact that C-peptide assays were already being used in clinical practice. Thus, it was not a case of waiting for standardization to occur before an assay can be used for patient care. Indeed, given the level of effort required for full harmonization, it is not likely that any new assays would ever be introduced into practice if they must first undergo a full program of formal harmonization. The lessons learned from the C-peptide story are also applicable to less formalized harmonization efforts, differing mainly in degree and scope when applied to formal versus less-formal harmonization efforts.

ROLE OF PROFICIENCY TESTING

Although this article has emphasized the need for more extensive harmonization efforts, one should not overlook the role of proficiency testing. It is best to think of proficiency testing programs not as full harmonization programs in and of themselves, but rather as programs to maintain harmony between methods within a harmonization effort. In many countries, proficiency testing programs have regulatory authority. If a laboratory consistently fails proficiency testing for a given analyte it may result in the laboratory being unable to offer that test.

Furthermore, as discussed later in this article, the CDC hormone standardization program includes a proficiency testing program for steroid hormones.[14] This could provide a model for the role of proficiency testing in harmonization and standardization efforts for protein assays by LC-MS/MS.

There are at least 3 aspects of proficiency testing that interact with each other to affect harmonization. One addresses the issue of whether methods themselves agree with each other (harmonization between methods). Another is whether different laboratories that run the same method produce results that agree with each other (harmonization within a peer group). The third is whether the methods agree with a well-defined and agreed-on standard of absolute accuracy (standardization). To understand the role of proficiency testing in practical harmonization efforts, one must keep these 3 aspects in mind.

One significant question that needs to be considered, even at the present stage of historical development, is whether it is sufficient to seek harmony between the methods in a proficiency testing program, or should the program aspire to the higher goal of absolute accuracy. An anecdote from the realm of LC-MS/MS testing of small molecules can help frame the issue. Some years back, one of the laboratories performing LC-MS/MS testing of metanephrines was consistently failing proficiency testing within its peer group. That proficiency testing program was based on harmony between laboratories, not absolute accuracy. An investigation showed that the laboratory that was consistently failing proficiency testing was also the laboratory that was consistently producing the more accurate results.[15] Therefore, when constructing or participating in a proficiency testing program, it is important to consider the goals of the program. Is it to be harmony-based or accuracy-based, and how are the results to be evaluated to ensure the best patient care?

The commutability issue is also applicable in proficiency testing programs, particularly in cases in which samples may be unstable. In those cases, the proficiency samples may be designed to improve stability, which can sometimes have the side effect of making the samples less like natural patient samples and therefore at greater risk of being noncommutable.

METHOD CONSIDERATIONS

In general, the methods used for analysis fundamentally affect the prospects for successful harmonization, and assays using LC-MS/MS for protein analysis are no different. As mentioned earlier, some MS methods for protein analysis have demonstrated good agreement even in the absence of rigorous use of reference materials. This is related to the fact that direct analysis of protein fragments broadens the options for first principle approaches to quantitative analysis.

In contrast to immunologic methods, in which access to selected epitopes is governed by immunoreactivity of the organism selected for antibody production, a diverse range of proteotypic peptides can be accessed based on the requirements of the method. In many cases, preanalytical conditions can be finely tuned to derive the measurement from peptides that demonstrate optimal properties for analysis, as well as containing specific amino acid polymorphisms, posttranslational modifications, or cleavages, as needed. This process is not without constraints. It is recognized that some proteins/peptides present biophysical and biochemical challenges that reduce their value for analytical characterization, and there remain proteins that are refractory to elements of the required preanalytical sample preparation.

A few things that should be considered when designing and validating a method include whether to use a top-down method (MS method of a whole protein, possibly including MS/MS), a bottom-up method (digesting the protein and detecting specific peptides as surrogates for the target protein), which peptides to target in a digestion-based method, how many peptides to target in the method, what calibrators to use, choice of internal standards, and the quality of the LC separation necessary for a successful LC-MS/MS–based method. All of these things ultimately affect the prospects for successful method harmonization. An example of a decision matrix for calibrator selection is given in **Fig. 5**.

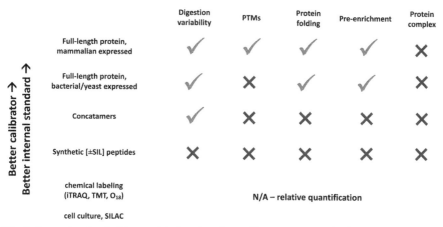

Fig. 5. Example of a decision matrix for choosing calibrators. Green check marks indicate an analytical consideration for which the given calibrator accounts for a given source of bias. iTRAQ, Isobaric tags for relative and absolute quantitation; N/A, not applicable; 18O-Oxygen-18; PTM, Post translational modification; SILAC, Stable Isotope Labeling by/with Amino acids in Cell culture; SIL,stable isotope labeled; TMT, Tandem Mass Tag.

LITERATURE REVIEW/BIBLIOGRAPHY

Laboratory assays commonly provide results for 700 or more types of quantities, with varying degrees of metrological traceability.[16] Primary reference measurement procedures (RMPs) *and* primary reference materials are available for 25 to 30 (conservatively) types of quantities linking these assays traceable to the SI. Reference materials without associated RMPs can be found for more than 300 types of quantities. RMPs without primary reference materials are less common (~30 quantities). Regrettably, most current laboratory assays (>300) are run exclusively using "in-house" calibrators and measurement procedures.

Implementing a successful assay harmonization effort should be considered compulsory to ensure the comparability of patient results.[17] However, there are currently relatively few examples of successful harmonization efforts. That number is growing, largely reflecting the implementation of electronic health records by physicians and hospitals,[18] and thanks to government directives such as the European Union's In Vitro Diagnostic Directive[19] or regulations such as the Food and Drug Administration's Clinical Laboratory Improvement Amendments guidance.[20] Independent bodies, such as AACC/International Federation of Clinical Chemistry and Laboratory Medicine (IFCC) and Joint Committee for Traceability in Laboratory Medicine, World Health Organization (WHO), Clinical and Laboratory Standards Institute, as well as national entities like NIST and National Institutes of Health (NIH)/CDC, are leading the international harmonization effort. Included among the harmonization success stories to date are efforts such as the CDC's HoSt program, which is focused on serum hormones like thyroid-stimulating hormone,[21] estradiol and, testosterone,[22] and the NIH/Office of Dietary Supplements Vitamin D Standardization Program.[4,23] Other organizations have also led efforts to create international standards for measurands like serum immunoglobulin E[24] (College of American Pathologists (CAP), WHO), free thyroxine,[25] triiodothyronine[26] (IFCC), and for lipid function tests such as cholesterol[27] (NIST), and kidney function measurement of serum creatinine[28] (NIST). In some cases, atypically, harmonization of clinical assays results from only a single manufacturer producing a test specific for a given measurand (N terminal-proBNP, cardiac troponin T)[5,29] (Roche Diagnostics, Risch-Rotkreuz, Switzerland).

The International Consortium for Harmonization of Clinical Laboratory Results provides an updated resource summarizing the measurand harmonization activities ongoing throughout the world (http://www.harmonization.net/measurands). Practical approaches to harmonizing routine laboratory methods have been described.[30,31] Useful resources are sufficiently available for understanding past and ongoing assay harmonization efforts, for establishing traceability of results, and for understanding commutability of standards.[14] Harmonization of laboratory testing requires cooperation from international stakeholder communities, including clinicians, medical device manufacturers, and standards, metrology, governmental, and professional organizations, and others.[32]

The CDC hormone standardization program provides a useful model that could be emulated for protein measurements by LC-MS/MS.[33] This program focuses on 4 main components: (1) developing and implementing reference methods, calibrated using "pure compound" hormones, (2) establishing an assay and laboratory calibration program to (among other functions) ensure the calibration does not change over time, (3) working with proficiency testing companies to develop laboratory surveys to assess and improve the measurement of targeted hormones, and (4) collaborating with professional organizations and institutions to develop training and education materials.

SUMMARY

Assay harmonization is a collaborative effort typically requiring long-term commitment, technical expertise, and financial resources. Achieving this significant goal is a worthwhile investment. As a practical matter, this article advocates a multistep approach to harmonization of LC-MS/MS–based protein assays, starting with small-scale preliminary harmonization efforts, culminating with full-scale harmonization efforts that follow the harmonization roadmap. The ultimate goal of fully standardized assays may remain elusive for quite some time. This approach will likely be done on an analyte-by-analyte basis in most cases, although there may sometimes be potential for multiplexing multiple.

LC-MS/MS is beginning to be applied to the analysis of proteins for diagnostic purposes. The high specificity of LC-MS/MS brings with it advantages and opportunities for improved analytical performance for improved diagnostic performance and better patient care; however, in some cases, this high degree of specificity can also be a risk if it targets clinically irrelevant forms. Proper assay development remains the key to avoiding this type of failure.

Harmonization between methods has received greater emphasis in recent years, and formalized approaches for method harmonization have been developed. However, relatively few clinical analytes have been harmonized or standardized to the high level required under these schemes. In this respect, MS-based methods are still at an early stage, possibly even lagging behind more established methods in the clinical laboratory. To our knowledge, no protein assays based on LC-MS/MS have been rigorously harmonized or standardized to date.

Nevertheless, as clinical laboratory scientists, we must diligently work toward harmonization of our LC-MS/MS methods, even if it is not yet practical to fully implement the most rigorous harmonization protocols that are being developed. We have presented the example of a preliminary Tg harmonization study as a prototype for bootstrapping the harmonization process; that is, early efforts to bring methods into harmonization before the implementation of the highest level of harmonization, and we have extracted lessons taken from that study and used them to outline a general approach for early-stage harmonization efforts.

Also presented are technical aspects of MS in relation to how they may affect the harmonization process and a short review of some of the relevant literature.

ACKNOWLEDGMENTS

Helpful discussions with Geoffrey Rule are gratefully acknowledged.

REFERENCES

1. AACC POSITION STATEMENT - Harmonization of clinical laboratory test results [Web site], 2013. Available at: https://www.harmonization.net/media/1087/aacc_harmonization_position_statement_2013.pdf. Accessed June 7, 2018.
2. Greg Miller W, Myers GL, Lou Gantzer M, et al. Roadmap for harmonization of clinical laboratory measurement procedures. Clin Chem 2011;57(8):1108–17.
3. Vesper HW, Botelho JC, Wang Y. Challenges and improvements in testosterone and estradiol testing. Asian J Androl 2014;16(2):178–84.
4. Phinney KW, Sempos CT, Tai SS, et al. Baseline assessment of 25-Hydroxyvitamin D reference material and proficiency testing/external quality assurance material commutability: a vitamin D standardization program study. J AOAC Int 2017; 100(5):1288–93.
5. Saenger AK, Rodriguez-Fraga O, Ler R, et al. Specificity of B-type natriuretic peptide assays: cross-reactivity with different BNP, NT-proBNP, and proBNP peptides. Clin Chem 2017;63(1):351–8.
6. Kaufmann A, Butcher P, Maden K, et al. Are liquid chromatography/electrospray tandem quadrupole fragmentation ratios unequivocal confirmation criteria? Rapid Commun mass Spectrom 2009;23(7):985–98.
7. Wang J, Aubry A, Bolgar MS, et al. Effect of mobile phase pH, aqueous-organic ratio, and buffer concentration on electrospray ionization tandem mass spectrometric fragmentation patterns: implications in liquid chromatography/tandem mass spectrometric bioanalysis. Rapid Commun mass Spectrom 2010;24(22): 3221–9.
8. Nilsson G, Budd JR, Greenberg N, et al. IFCC working group recommendations for assessing commutability part 2: using the difference in bias between a reference material and clinical samples. Clin Chem 2018;64(3):455–64.
9. Miller WG, Schimmel H, Rej R, et al. IFCC working group recommendations for assessing commutability part 1: general experimental design. Clin Chem 2018; 64(3):447–54.
10. Budd JR, Weykamp C, Rej R, et al. IFCC working group recommendations for assessing commutability part 3: using the calibration effectiveness of a reference material. Clin Chem 2018;64(3):465–74.
11. Netzel BC, Grebe SK, Carranza Leon BG, et al. Thyroglobulin (Tg) testing revisited: Tg assays, Tgab assays, and correlation of results with clinical outcomes. J Clin Endocrinol Metab 2015;100(8):E1074–83.
12. Netzel BC, Grant RP, Hoofnagle AN, et al. First steps toward harmonization of LC-MS/MS thyroglobulin assays. Clin Chem 2016;62(1):297–9.
13. Little RR, Wielgosz RI, Josephs R, et al. Implementing a reference measurement system for c-peptide: successes and lessons learned. Clin Chem 2017;63(9):1447–56.
14. Prevention CfDCa. HoSt/VDSCP: standardization of measurement procedures. Laboratory Quality Assurance and Standardization Programs. 2017.
15. Singh RJ, Grebe SK, Yue B, et al. Precisely wrong? Urinary fractionated metanephrines and peer-based laboratory proficiency testing. Clin Chem 2005; 51(2):472–3 [discussion 473–4].

16. International Organization for Standardization (ISO). In vitro diagnostic medical devices – Measurement of quantities in biological samples – metrological traceability of values assigned to calibrators and control materials. ISO 17511:2003.

17. Panteghini M. Traceability, reference systems and result comparability. Clin Biochem Rev 2007;28(3):97–104.

18. Office-based Physician Electronic Health Record Adoption. Health IT Quick-Stat #50 2016; Health IT Quick-Stat #50. Available at: dashboard.healthit.gov/quickstats/pages/physician-ehr-adoption-trends.php. Accessed June 7, 2018.

19. Directive 98/79/EC of the European parliament and of the council of 27 October 1998 on in vitro diagnostic medical devices. Official Journal of the European Communities 1998;41(L 331).

20. US Food and Drug Administration (FDA), 2018. Clinical Laboratory Improvement Amendments (CLIA), Medical Devisces, IVD Regulatory Assistance. Available at: https://www.fda.gov/MedicalDevices/DeviceRegulationandGuidance/IVDRegulatory Assistance/ucm124105.htm. Accessed June 7, 2018.

21. Thienpont LM, Van Uytfanghe K, De Grande LAC, et al. Harmonization of serum thyroid-stimulating hormone measurements paves the way for the adoption of a more uniform reference interval. Clin Chem 2017;63(7): 1248–60.

22. Travison TG, Vesper HW, Orwoll E, et al. Harmonized reference ranges for circulating testosterone levels in men of four cohort studies in the United States and Europe. J Clin Endocrinol Metab 2017;102(4):1161–73.

23. Wise SA, Phinney KW, Tai SS, et al. Baseline assessment of 25-Hydroxyvitamin D assay performance: a Vitamin D standardization program (VDSP) interlaboratory comparison study. J AOAC Int 2017;100(5):1244–52.

24. Thorpe SJ, Heath A, Fox B, et al. The 3rd International Standard for serum IgE: international collaborative study to evaluate a candidate preparation. Clin Chem Lab Med 2014;52(9):1283–9.

25. Faix JD, Miller WG. Progress in standardizing and harmonizing thyroid function tests. Am J Clin Nutr 2016;104(Suppl 3):913s–7s.

26. Thienpont LM, Van Uytfanghe K, Beastall G, et al. Report of the IFCC working group for standardization of thyroid function tests; part 2: free thyroxine and free triiodothyronine. Clin Chem 2010;56(6):912–20.

27. Ellerbe P, Meiselman S, Sniegoski LT, et al. Determination of serum cholesterol by a modification of the isotope dilution mass spectrometric definitive method. Anal Chem 1989;61(15):1718–23.

28. Camara JE, Lippa KA, Duewer DL, et al. An international assessment of the metrological equivalence of higher-order measurement services for creatinine in serum. Anal Bioanal Chem 2012;403(2):527–35.

29. Januzzi JL, van Kimmenade R, Lainchbury J, et al. NT-proBNP testing for diagnosis and short-term prognosis in acute destabilized heart failure: an international pooled analysis of 1256 patients: the International Collaborative of NT-proBNP Study. Eur Heart J 2006;27(3):330–7.

30. Greaves RF. A guide to harmonisation and standardisation of measurands determined by liquid chromatography–tandem mass spectrometry in routine clinical biochemistry. Clin Biochem Rev 2012;33(4):123–32.

31. Vesper HW, Myers GL, Miller WG. Current practices and challenges in the standardization and harmonization of clinical laboratory tests. Am J Clin Nutr 2016; 104(Suppl 3):907s–12s.

32. Tate JR, Johnson R, Barth J, et al. Harmonization of laboratory testing—current achievements and future strategies. Clin Chim Acta 2014;432:4–7.
33. Centers for Disease Control and Prevention (CDC), 2018. Standardizing Hormone Measurements Program, Web site. Available at: https://www.cdc.gov/labstandards/pdf/hs/HoSt_Brochure.pdf. Accessed June 7, 2018.

Accreditation and Quality Assurance for Clinical Liquid Chromatography–Mass Spectrometry Laboratories

Kara L. Lynch, PhD

KEYWORDS

- Liquid chromatography mass spectrometry • Quality management system
- Quality control • Quality assurance • Clinical laboratory accreditation • CLSI C62A

KEY POINTS

- The 5 Clinical Laboratory Improvement Amendments' requirements for laboratory accreditation (facility administration, quality systems, proficiency testing, personnel, and inspection) apply to laboratories performing liquid chromatography–tandem mass spectrometry (LC-MS/MS) testing.
- Although there is sufficient guidance on LC-MS/MS method validation and verification, only Clinical and Laboratory Standards Institute C62A provides some guidance on best practices for quality assurance and postimplementation monitoring.
- Quality-assurance monitoring for LC-MS/MS testing should be proactive rather than reactive and should monitor the entire testing process, including preanalytical, analytical, and postanalytical.
- An LC-MS/MS quality-assurance plan should cover overall batch review parameters, individual peak review parameters, system and reagent changes, and assessment of long-term accuracy.

INTRODUCTION

The ability to accurately identify and quantify an analyte with high sensitivity and specificity by the use of selective reactive monitoring has been the driving force for the adoption of liquid chromatography (LS)–mass spectrometry (MS) in the clinical laboratory. The field has seen a significant increase in the number of clinical LC-MS applications in the past decade, and more clinical laboratories continue to adopt the technology for diagnostic testing. Despite its widespread use, there are very few quantitative LC-MS assays approved by the US Food and Drug Administration (FDA); all other assays fall under the

Disclosure Statement: Nothing to disclose.
Department of Laboratory Medicine, Clinical Laboratory, Zuckerberg San Francisco General Hospital, University of California San Francisco, 1001 Potrero Avenue. Building. 5 2M, San Francisco, CA 94110, USA
E-mail address: kara.lynch@ucsf.edu

Clin Lab Med 38 (2018) 515–526
https://doi.org/10.1016/j.cll.2018.05.002
0272-2712/18/© 2018 Elsevier Inc. All rights reserved.

FDA classification of laboratory developed test (LDT). An LDT is defined as an in vitro diagnostic test that is designed, manufactured, validated, and used within a single laboratory. Therefore, no 2 LC-MS methods for the same analyte are alike. Despite the variability in the analytical methods used across laboratories, all clinical laboratories are subject to regulations under CLIA and are held to the highest standard of quality. Although there is sufficient guidance on LC-MS method validation and verification, only the Clinical and Laboratory Standards Institute's (CLSI) guidance document C62-A provides some guidance on best practices for quality assurance (QA) and postimplementation method monitoring.[1] QA monitoring for LC–tandem MS (MS/MS) testing should be proactive rather than reactive and should monitor the entire testing process: preanalytical, analytical, and postanalytical. An LC-MS/MS QA plan should cover overall batch review parameters, individual peak review parameters, system and reagent changes, and assessment of long-term accuracy. This article discusses the CLIA's regulations as they apply to LC-MS/MS–based testing and reviews available guidelines for LC-MS/MS QA monitoring.

LIQUID CHROMATOGRAPHY–TANDEM MASS SPECTROMETRY LABORATORY ACCREDITATION

Most clinical laboratories implementing LC-MS testing do so in the context of an existing accredited laboratory. The requirements for accreditation should, thus, be familiar and similar to other laboratory sections. All clinical laboratories in the United States performing diagnostic testing on human specimens operate under direct federal regulation by the Department of Health and Human Services, Center for Medicare and Medicaid Services (CMS). Diagnostic laboratories are subject to the Clinical Laboratory Improvement Amendments of 1988 (CLIA or CLIA 1988).[2] CLIA definition of a laboratory is "a facility for the biological, microbiological, serological, chemical, immunohematological, hematological, biophysical, cytological, pathological, or other examination of material derived from the human body for the purpose of providing information for the diagnosis, prevention, or treatment of any disease or impairment of, or the assessment of the health of, human beings." CLIA requires clinical laboratories to be either CLIA exempt or hold a CLIA certificate. CLIA-exempt laboratories primarily include research, forensic, federal, and Substance Abuse and Mental Health Services Administration laboratories. Laboratories that preform high-complexity testing, such as LC-MS, require a CLIA certificate of accreditation. The CMS grants private nonprofit accreditation agencies deemed status for accrediting clinical laboratories. The requirements of the accreditation agency must be equal to, or more stringent than, the CLIA's requirements. Common nonprofit accreditation agencies with deemed status that inspect clinical LC-MS laboratories include COLA (formerly Commission on Laboratory Accreditation), the College of American Pathologists (CAP), and The Joint Commission (TJC).

The following sections discuss the CLIA's 5 requirements for clinical laboratory accreditation as they pertain to laboratories preforming LC-MS methods. Where relevant, each section highlights the available guidelines and best practices for routine LC-MS testing. The 5 requirements for laboratory accreditation include facility administration, quality systems, participation in proficiency testing, personnel, and inspection.

FACILITY ADMINISTRATION: CLINICAL LABORATORY IMPROVEMENT AMENDMENTS REQUIREMENT 1

CLIA requires the implementation of written policies and procedures that ensure a safe working environment for the testing preformed. Safety procedures must be accessible and observed to provide protection from electrical, physical, chemical, biochemical, and biological hazards. In addition to the CLIA's regulations regarding laboratory safety, clinical laboratories are subject to several Occupational Safety and Health Administration (OSHA), federal, state, and local safety regulations. OHSA regulation 29 Code of Federal Regulations (CFR) 1910 covers topics such as air contamination, general housekeeping, sanitation/waste disposal, standards for hazard communication, personal protective equipment, and exposure to blood-borne pathogens and hazardous chemicals. Requirements for occupational injury and illness recording and reporting are defined in OHSA regulation 29 CFR 1904 and 1952. Other regulations worth noting include the Medical Waste Tracking Act of 1988, the Health Insurance Portability and Accountability Act of 1996, and subsequent regulations that include protection of health information and electronic medical records.

Clinical laboratories are also subject to the regulations governing the retention of records. Records that must be retained for 2 years include test requisitions, test procedures, analytical systems records (quality control [QC], patient test records, instrument printouts), records of test system performance, proficiency testing records, and quality system assessment records and test reports. These records may be retained in electronic format providing that they can be accessed and printed in their original format as appropriate or on request during an accreditation inspection.

QUALITY SYSTEMS: CLINICAL LABORATORY IMPROVEMENT AMENDMENTS REQUIREMENT 2

A quality management system (QMS) encompasses the policies and procedures that enable a laboratory to meet its stated quality goals. CLIA states "Each laboratory that performs non-waived testing must establish and maintain written policies and procedures that implement and monitor a quality system for all phases of the total testing process (that is, preanalytical, analytical, and postanalytical) as well as general laboratory systems. ... This must include a quality assessment component that ensures continuous improvement of the laboratory's performance and services through ongoing monitoring that identifies, evaluates and resolves problems." The CLSI has developed several guidelines to help guide the design of an effective QMS for routine testing using FDA-approved methods. Despite the fact that LC-MS methods are primarily laboratory-developed tests that are not FDA-approved methods, the CLSI's QMS guidelines are still valuable resources for clinical LC-MS laboratories. Of particular interest are CLSI QMS01, *Quality Management System: A Model for Laboratory Services*; CLSI QMS06, *Quality Management System: Continual Improvement*; and QMS12, *Development and Use of Quality Indicators for Process Improvement of Monitoring of Laboratory Quality*.[3–5]

There are 2 critical components of a QMS: QC and QA. The CLSI provides specific guidelines for performing QC testing in CLSI-EP23, *Laboratory Quality Control Based on Risk Management*.[6] However, there are only 2 CLSI guidance documents primarily focused on the use of LC-MS in clinical laboratories and only one provides information relating to QA practices. CLSI C50-A, *Mass Spectrometry in the Clinical Laboratory: General Principles and Guidance; Approved Guideline*, provides a general understanding of MS and the principles that dictate its application in the clinical laboratory but falls short of offering a systematic approach for method development, validation, and postimplementation monitoring.[7] In 2014, the CLSI published CLSI C62-A, *Liquid-Chromatography-Mass Spectrometry Methods; Approved Guidelines*.[8] CLSI C62-A outlines best practices for assay development, preverification, verification, quality assessment, and postimplementation monitoring. It was the first guideline to include information specific to QC and QA for quantitative LC-MS testing. The recommended guidelines pertaining to QA for LC-MS are discussed next.

Quality Assurance

Liquid chromatography–tandem mass spectrometry method development requirements

The first step to quality for LC-MS/MS is the development and verification of an accurate and robust method. For this, there are several established guidelines, such as CLSI-C62-A, the FDA's "Guidance for Industry: Bioanalytical Method Validation," the European Medicines Agency's (EMA) "Guideline on Bioanalytical Method Validation," and the Scientific Working Group for Forensic Toxicology "Standard Practices for Method Validation."[1,8–10] Also, the CLIA's regulations ("Subpart K, Quality Systems for Nonwaived Testing") specify requirements for establishment and verification of performance specifications for laboratory-developed tests. These requirements include accuracy, precision, analytical sensitivity, analytical specificity to include interfering substances, reportable range of test results for the test system, reference intervals, and any other performance characteristic required for test performance. When laboratories are inspected for accreditation, an inspector is required to review the validation of all new methods to ensure that it is adequate and meets all regulatory requirements. Details regarding the best practices for LC-MS method validation are discussed in Uttam Garg's article, "Special Considerations for LCMSMS Method Development," in this issue.

Quality-assurance monitoring

Although there is ample guidance for LC-MS method development and validation, surprisingly only CLSI-C62-A provides best practices for QA and postimplementation monitoring. However, the QA guidelines typically advise that "an acceptable range/tolerance should be established during method development (by the laboratory)"[1] suggesting that each method will call for its own quality measures. Despite the lack of literature available on what constitutes a QMS for LC-MS/MS testing, some standard quality measures are often used by clinical laboratories using LC-MS/MS. An LC-MS/MS QA plan should cover every peak, batch, system and reagent changes, and assessment of long-term accuracy.

System suitability test The key to a good QA plan is to catch system issues before they affect routine testing. Many laboratories use system suitability testing to monitor instrument performance. A system suitability test (SST) uses a reference solution to verify performance of the LC-MS/MS analytical system. This reference solution contains the nonextracted analytes and internal standards for a given method and should be evaluated after instrument maintenance, a power outage, break in instrument vacuum, instrument tuning/calibration, and before sample analysis. According to CLSI-C62-A, acceptance criteria for the SST should be set for variables, such as retention time, peak height and width, ion ratio, and signal to noise (S/N) ratio. CLSI-C62-A also recommends that a minimum of 3 samples should be evaluated before batch analysis and after instrument maintenance. It also suggests that the ion ratio of replicates should have a coefficient of variation (CV) less than 6% and the S/N ratio be greater than 10:1 for the SST at the extracted lower limit of the measuring interval (LLMI). **Table 1** highlights some possible patterns and trends that may be observed when performing an SST and the possible causes of these trends.

Batch and peak review Monitoring sample analysis performance, which is the largest component of an LC-MS/MS QA plan, can be subdivided into 2 categories: overall

Table 1
Liquid chromatography–tandem mass spectrometry quality-assurance parameters

Parameter to Monitor	CLSI-C62A Recommendation	Possible Patterns/ Trends	Possible Causes
SST	• Acceptance criteria should be set for variables, such as Rt, peak height and width, ion ratio, and S/N ratio • Minimum of 3 samples should be evaluated before batch analysis and after instrument maintenance • Ion ratio of replicates should have a CV <6% • S/N ratio should be >10:1 for SST at extracted LLMI	• Shift in Rt or RRt • Peak asymmetry • Change in peak intensity • Detection of additional peaks • Ion ratio change • Decrease in S/N ratio	• Mobile phase change/ degradation/evaporation • LC-MS system malfunction/failure • LC column change/ deterioration • Temperature fluctuations • New interferent in system • MS maintenance/ cleaning required
Calibrator accuracy and calibration curve slope	• Allowable bias should be ±15% for all calibrators greater than the LLMI and ±20% for LLMI • Calibration slope should be $r^2 \geq 0.995$	• Nonlinearity or change in appropriateness of linear fit • Unacceptable bias for one calibrator or multiple calibrators	• Calibrator deterioration • Loss of detector sensitivity • Insufficient volume of injection • Pipetting/sample preparation error • Poor preparative recovery
Internal standard (IS) peak area	• Acceptable range for IS peak area should be defined during method validation • IS peak areas should be comparable across calibrators and controls in the same run	• Sporadic IS shift throughout run or for individual samples • Gradual shift in IS peak area • Drastic shift in IS peak area (within or between batches)	• Instrument drift/charging • Poor preparative recovery • Failure to precisely aliquot IS • Unacceptable ionization suppression/enhancement from matrix effects • Insufficient volume of injection • Degradation of IS
QC	• A minimum of 3 QC concentrations should be tested in duplicate per batch • Acceptable QC mean and SD should be established by repetitive analysis, not manufacturer provided ranges • New lots of QC should be evaluated according to CLSI-C24 • All failed QC must be investigated and corrective action documented	• Random QC failure in batch • Gradual QC shift over time • Drastic QC shift	• QC deterioration • Loss of detector sensitivity • Insufficient volume of injection • Pipetting/sample preparation error • Poor preparative recovery

(continued on next page)

Table 1
(continued)

Parameter to Monitor	CLSI-C62A Recommendation	Possible Patterns/ Trends	Possible Causes
Analyte Rt and/or RRt to internal standard	• Rt or RRt for sample should be within ±2.5% of the mean Rt/ RRt of the calibrators in the same batch (and between batches)	• Sporadic shift in Rt or RRt • Gradual shift in Rt or RRt • Drastic shift in Rt or RRt (within or between batches)	• Mobile phase change/ degradation/evaporation • LC pump malfunction/ failure • LC column change/ deterioration • Temperature fluctuations
Ion ratio	• Acceptable range for ion ratio should be determined during method validation • Mean ratio of the calibrators should not alter significantly within or between runs • If signal of qualifier ion is >50% that of the quantifier ion, the ion ratio in the patient samples should be ±20% from that of the mean ratio of the calibrators	• Ion ratio outside of acceptable range for individual patient sample • Significant change in ion ratio mean between runs • Ion ratio outside of acceptable range for samples with analytes near the LLMI	• Integration failure of precursor or product ion • Interfering substance in an individual patient sample • Reagent or system change resulting in new interfering substance throughout a batch • Loss in assay sensitivity resulting in inadequate signal for qualifier ion

Abbreviations: Rt, retention time; RRt, relative retention time; SD, standard deviation.

Adapted from Lynch KL. LC-MS/MS quality assurance in production. Clinical Laboratory News 2017;43(5):28–9. Copyright AACC, used *with permission.*

batch review parameters and individual peak review parameters. The first focuses on calibration curve acceptance, internal standard (IS) recovery throughout the batch, and QC acceptance.

Calibration CLSI-C62-A, FDA, and EMA all recommend that a calibration curve contain a blank, zero, and 6 to 8 calibration standards prepared in the same biological matrix as the samples, placed at the LLMI, upper limit of the measuring interval (ULMI), and any medically relevant decision point within the analytical measurable interval (AMI). When generating the calibration curve, laboratories must use the same fit (linear or quadratic) and the same weighting factors (eg, $1/x$ or $1/x^2$) as defined in their method validation. A change in the appropriateness of the fit should prompt the laboratory to investigate the root cause. With the curve established, calibrator accuracy should be ±15% for all points except the lowest calibrator (±20%). In addition, the curve slope should be r^2 0.995 or greater. The guidelines from the FDA and EMA state that only 75% of calibrators must meet allowable bias, which is much more lenient than CLSI-C62-A.

Internal standard peak area According to CLSI-C62-A, the acceptance range for the IS peak area should be defined during method validation. The IS peak area should be comparable across calibrators and controls in the same analytical run. Changes in IS recovery within and between batches may indicate potential problems at multiple points in the analytical process, including instrument drift and charging, insufficient injection volume, poor sample preparative recovery, and, most importantly, unacceptable ionization suppression or enhancement in an individual sample.

Quality control Although laboratories should use standard clinical laboratory QC practice for LC-MS/MS methods, according to CLSI-C62-A, the number of QC samples analyzed during a batch should represent at least 5% of the total number of patient samples or at least 6 total (3 concentrations analyzed in duplicate). It is suggested that the 3 concentrations of the QC samples should include 3 times the LLMI, midrange, and near the ULMI. The acceptable QC mean and standard deviation should be established by repetitive analysis and not by the manufacturer's provided ranges. New lots of QC should be evaluated according to CLSI-C24, "Quality Control for Quantitative Measurement."[11] All failed QC samples must be investigated and corrective action documented.

Analyte peak review Once a laboratory deems a batch acceptable, individual samples/peaks must meet preestablished ranges for ion ratios and retention time (Rt) and/or relative Rt (RRt) to the internal standard. CLSI-C62-A recommends that the Rt or RRt for samples should be within $\pm 2.5\%$ of the mean Rt/RRt of the calibrators in the same batch (and between batches). Shifts in the Rt or RRt within or between batches, whether they be sporadic, gradual, or drastic, can indicate several potential issues primarily with the LC system. These issues include a potential mobile phase change, degradation, or evaporation. They can also indicate LC pump malfunction or LC column change or deterioration. Temperature changes within the LC could also result in Rt or RRt shifts.

Laboratories should calculate a mean ion ratio (qualifying ion peak area/quantifying ion peak area) for the calibrators in each batch, which should not vary significantly within or between runs. CLSI-C62-A specifies that if the signal of the qualifier ion is greater than 50% that of the quantifier ion, the ion ratio in a patient sample should be within 20% from the mean ratio of the standards. A failed ion ratio in a patient sample suggests a possible peak integration failure, loss of assay sensitivity, and/or interfering substance. Interferents should not alter the calculated concentration of analyte or the ion ratio.

System and reagent changes LC-MS/MS laboratories use several consumable materials and liquid reagents for LC-MS/MS methods. These materials may include sample preparation reagents, mobile phases, analytical columns, calibration standards, QC material, and internal standard, to name a few. Some of these reagents may be prepared manually because the LC-MS/MS methods are laboratory-developed tests. CLSI-C62-A states that all new lots of consumables and reagents must be compared with current lots. For new calibrators and controls, they must be run as unknowns to establish set points. Patient samples should be evaluated with both lots of calibrators to ensure that the results are consistent. For a change in the analytical column, CLSI-C62-A states that a minimum of 5 patient samples must be evaluated with the new analytical column and compared with the results for the old analytical column. For patient comparison samples, acceptability criteria should be based on preestablished acceptability criteria and method performance requirements. The concentrations of the patient samples used to verify a new column or reagent change should span the AMI.

Long-term accuracy Monitoring assay performance over time is essential to ensure quality. An LC-MS/MS QA plan should include procedures for daily, weekly, and periodic maintenance of the analytical instrumentation. The manufacturer's recommendations for instrument maintenance should serve as the starting point for clinical laboratories; however, most manufacturers only provide minimal recommendations for weekly and periodic maintenance. As a laboratory becomes more familiar with their instrument system and assays, additional maintenance items may be added to the maintenance schedule in order to circumvent issues before they arise. Maintenance should be performed at a specified frequency and documented. Completion of daily, weekly, and periodic maintenance should be monitored using a checklist that includes the signature of the technologist performing the maintenance and the date of completion. Daily maintenance should be performed on all days of testing before patient samples are analyzed. Typical maintenance activities may include cleaning the curtain plate and source, cleaning the first quadrupole, checking the oil level of the roughing pump, checking the column pressure, and monitoring the number of injections on the analytical column. Specific maintenance requirements will vary from instrument to instrument. The periodic maintenance is typically performed under a service contract at a 6-month interval for the LC and MS. For the MS, this scheduled maintenance usually includes instrument calibration and tuning. This maintenance involves assigning accurate mass values to specific ion peaks and adjusting instrument parameters, such as voltages and gas flow, to optimize peak intensities. CLSI-C62-A specifies that each laboratory must establish the acceptability criteria for allowable total ion count, ion intensity, peak resolution, and mass shift. Mass calibration should also be performed or verified after major maintenance, environmental change, instrument failure, or when the instrument vacuum is compromised. For the LC, the periodic maintenance using involves cleaning the system and replacing parts that undergo significant wear and tear to ensure the system is in optimal operating condition.

In addition to instrument maintenance, ensuring long-term accuracy includes specific instrument/assay verifications every 6 months. As with all clinical laboratory quantitative assays, verifying assay linearity, accuracy, and instrument correlations (if the laboratory is using more than one instrument for the same method) are not only required but key to providing quality results. Verification of the linearity of the assay is typically referred to as calibration verification. Materials of known concentration are tested in the same manner as patient specimens to assure the test system is accurately measuring samples throughout the reportable range.

CLSI-C62-A strongly recommends that periodic accuracy monitoring be performed every 6 months. If certified, commutable reference materials are available; the laboratory should validate the traceability of calibrator values for in-house prepared calibrators or for commercial calibrators that are not traceable to a National Institute of Standards and Technology (NIST) or Joint Committee for Traceability in Laboratory Medicine (JCTLM)–listed reference measurement procedure. If feasible, the use of calibrators with value assignments traceable to NIST- or JCTLM-listed reference method procedures is strongly encouraged. More information on traceability and method standardization can be found in CLSI EP32.[12] When more than one analytical system is used to report out the same test, it is a regulatory requirement to show correlation between the instruments every 6 months. According to CLSI C62-A, acceptability criteria should be based on method performance criteria and clinical use of the results. A set of patient samples should be evaluated on both instruments to ensure that they provide equivalent results.

PROFICIENCY TESTING: CLINICAL LABORATORY IMPROVEMENT AMENDMENTS REQUIREMENT 3

CLIA regulations mandate proficiency testing for regulated analytes. Some analytes measured by LDTs using LC-MS/MS are classified as regulated analytes, whereas others are considered nonregulated. Regardless of classification by CLIA, accreditation programs, such as CAP, require proficiency testing of most nonregulated analytes as well. Proficiency testing programs are available for common analytes by subscription, with challenges including 5 samples provided 3 times a year. A score of 80% is required for successful proficiency testing. The laboratory must have a successful score on 2 of 3 consecutive proficiency testing events. For many analytes measured by MS, there may be no formal proficiency testing program available. For these analytes, alternative means of proficiency testing must be established. Approaches to alternative proficiency testing include (1) measurement of assayed materials such as NIST standards, (2) comparison of split sample measurements with other laboratories, and (3) comparison with an alternative measurement method. It is the responsibility of the laboratory director to specify the frequency of alternative proficiency testing and the acceptance criteria for the results comparison. Evaluation and corrective action for failed proficiency testing and alternative method performance assessment is required for both regulated and nonregulated analytes. There must be evidence of review of proficiency testing reports by the laboratory director or designee. Evaluations must determine the likely cause of the failed sample analysis, the corrective action taken, and determination of whether patients' results could have been affected. CLSI QMS24 provides detailed instructions on how to use proficiency testing to improve quality in the clinical laboratory.[13]

PERSONNEL: CLINICAL LABORATORY IMPROVEMENT AMENDMENTS REQUIREMENT 4

The CLIA's regulations outline the qualifications and responsibilities for the laboratory director, technical consultants, clinical consultants, technical supervisors, general supervisors, and testing personnel. CLIA 1988, Subpart L lists the 15 responsibilities of the laboratory director, some of which can be delegated to a designee and others that cannot. A competency assessment of all technical staff is required for each test that the individual is approved by the laboratory director to perform. Assessment must occur semiannually during the first year of testing and annually thereafter. The CLIA's regulations require evaluation of 6 elements:

1. Direct observation of routine patient test performance, including patient preparation, if applicable, specimen handling, processing, and testing
2. Monitoring the recording and reporting of test results
3. Review of intermediate test results or worksheets, QC records, proficiency testing results, and preventative maintenance records
4. Direct observation of performance of instrument maintenance and function
5. Assessment of test performance through testing previously analyzed specimens, internal blind testing samples, or external proficiency testing samples
6. Assessment of problem-solving skills

   Laboratories must design competency assessment programs for each of the assays performed by MS and maintain all records of completion for each of the required elements. Given the complexity of MS methods, the competency assessment may be very involved in order to evaluate the competency for all 6 elements throughout all phases of the testing process.

INSPECTION: CLINICAL LABORATORY IMPROVEMENT AMENDMENTS REQUIREMENT 5

All CLIA-certified nonwaived laboratories require a biennial on-site inspection. The inspection may be performed by the CMS or an agency granted deemed status by the CMS for CLIA accreditation. As mentioned earlier, common nonprofit accreditation agencies with deemed status that inspect clinical LC-MS laboratories include COLA (formerly Commission on Laboratory Accreditation), CAP, and TJC.

For laboratory inspections through CAP, checklists are followed by the inspectors to cover all regulations. General checklists cover aspects of method validation; however, there are only a few checklist elements specifically targeted to the operation of LC-MS/MS assays in the clinical laboratory.[14] The first, CHM.18400, states that there must be written procedures for operation and calibration of the mass spectrometer. Specifically, MS tuning should occur according to the manufacturer's recommendations. For LC-MS/MS testing, this usually occurs at least every 6 months during the scheduled preventative maintenance. The tuning records must be maintained. Second, CHM.18600 specifies that the identification criteria for MS/MS must be validated and recorded. Specifically, 2 multiple reaction monitoring transitions (and multiple reaction monitoring ratio) should be monitored for each reportable analyte and one transition monitored for all internal standards. A specified Rt or RRt to the internal standard is also typically used as an additional identification criterion. Last, CHM.18825 states that there must be a record of assessment of matrix effects in LC-MS test development; CHM.18850 states that the laboratory must evaluate for possible ion suppression or enhancement in patient samples during routine testing. For specific information regarding appropriate experiments to preform to evaluate matrix effects during method validation, please see Uttam Garg's article, "25-Hydroxyvitamin D Testing: Immunoassays versus Tandem Mass Spectrometry," in this issue. For CHM.18850, it is specified that routine monitoring of the signal intensity of internal standards is an effective way to recognize signal suppression in a single patient sample, due to unexpected interfering components of the matrix.

In 2017, TJC implemented revisions to their standards and added 8 elements of performance related to the use of MS in the laboratory. These elements can be found in QSA.06.04.05 and are as follows:

QSA.06.04.05: The laboratory has written QC and testing procedures for MS that address the following:

1. The use of calibrators or QC materials with each batch of patient samples prepared for analysis
2. Extraction and use of control materials that challenge each step of the testing process
3. Criteria and frequency for establishing mass calibration and optimum performance
4. The detection and evaluation of carryover
5. For quantitative tests, an established reportable range and limit of detection
6. Establishment and validation of identification criteria for the specific technique applied (for example, LC-MS vs gas chromatography-MS)
7. Evaluation, reduction, and monitoring of matrix effects and ion suppression included in LC-MS
8. Procedures for MS followed by the laboratory

Like all laboratory tests, it is imperative to have written procedure manuals for all aspects of the testing process. These procedures must include specimen requirements, test calculations and interpretation of results, calibration and calibration verification procedures, control procedures, and maintenance procedures, as discussed throughout this article. Following successful inspection and correction of any cited deficiencies, the CMS provides a Certificate of Accreditation. The CMS or the accreditation agency for the laboratory has the right to perform additional inspections if deemed necessary.

REGULATION OF LABORATORY DEVELOPED TESTS

Since 2010, the laboratory community has been awaiting impending federal regulations for LDTs. All clinical LC-MS methods, with the exception of a few FDA-approved kits, are classified as LDTs. The FDA has expressed concern regarding the quality and clinical validity of LDTs offered by commercial reference laboratories and hospital-based clinical laboratories. Currently, LDTs are regulated under CLIA; it is unclear whether the FDA will ever follow through on their decision to extend their regulatory oversight to include LDTs. In the future, it could be a requirement to register all LDTs with the FDA. Meeting FDA registration requirements for LDTs would significantly increase the regulatory burden for clinical MS laboratories. Although this increased regulatory enforcement has yet to be enacted or confirmed, clinical LC-MS laboratories should be aware of the potential changes and be prepared for a potential increase in the level and extent of regulation. In January of 2017, the FDA issued a discussion paper on LDTs.[15] The paper does not represent the formal position of the FDA nor is it enforceable. In short, the paper confirmed that the FDA will not be issuing final guidance on the oversight of LDTs at the request of various stakeholders to allow for further public discussion on an appropriate oversight approach and to give congressional authorizing committees the opportunity to develop a legislative solution.

SUMMARY

Comprehensive method validation and postimplementation monitoring of clinical LC-MS/MS methods are vital to providing quality diagnostic results. It is not uncommon for an LC-MS/MS method to not perform to specifications such that a laboratory cannot report results without extensive troubleshooting or instrument service. An intelligently designed QA plan that monitors the entire testing process can significantly cut down on the instrument and method downtime. Each individual method in any given laboratory may not meet consensus QA guidelines, as discussed in this article; however, this does not negate the fact that these parameters are still essential to monitor. Even though LC-MS/MS instrumentation and analytical methods are of high complexity and different from most standard laboratory methodologies that are FDA approved, LC-MS laboratories are still held to the same CLIA standards and must meet the CLIA's 5 requirements for accreditation: facility administration, quality systems, proficiency testing, personnel, and inspection. Currently, regulatory oversight of the LC-MS/MS method, specifically LDTs, is enacted through CLIA; however, the future could hold increased scrutiny by the FDA. Clinical LC-MS/MS laboratories should strive to provide the most accurate results through standardization efforts and quality monitoring. Although the CLSI C62-A provides some guidance on approaches to QA monitoring, it falls short of providing a systematic approach. The clinical LC-MS/MS community should continue to share ideas and work toward a common understanding of how to provide the highest level of quality for LC-MS/MS clinical diagnostic testing.

REFERENCES

1. Clinical and Laboratory Standards Institute (CLSI). Liquid chromatography-mass spectrometry methods; approved guideline (C62-A). Wayne (PA): Clinical and Laboratory Standards Institute (CLSI); 2014.
2. Centers for Medicare and Medicaid Services (CMS). Clinical laboratory improvement amendments (CLIA). Available at: https://www.cms.gov/Regulations-and-Guidance/Legislation/CLIA/index.html?redirect=/clia/

3. Clinical and Laboratory Standards Institute (CLSI). Quality management system: a model for laboratory services (QMS 01). 4th edition. Wayne (PA): Clinical and Laboratory Standards Institute (CLSI); 2011.

4. Clinical and Laboratory Standards Institute (CLSI). Quality management system: continual improvement (QMS 06). 3rd edition. Wayne (PA): Clinical and Laboratory Standards Institute (CLSI); 2011.

5. Clinical and Laboratory Standards Institute (CLSI). Development and use of quality indicators for process improvement and monitoring of laboratory quality (QMS 12). Wayne (PA): Clinical and Laboratory Standards Institute (CLSI); 2010.

6. Clinical and Laboratory Standards Institute (CLSI). Laboratory quality control based on risk management (EP23). Wayne (PA): Clinical and Laboratory Standards Institute (CLSI); 2011.

7. Clinical and Laboratory Standards Institute (CLSI). Mass spectrometry in the clinical laboratory: general principles and guidance (C50-A). Wayne (PA): Clinical and Laboratory Standards Institute (CLSI); 2007.

8. U.S Department of Health and Human Services, Food and Drug Administration, Center for Drug Evaluation and Research. Guidance for industry: bioanalytical method validation. 2001. Available at: https://www.fda.gov/downloads/Drugs/Guidance/ucm070107.pdf. Accessed April, 2018.

9. European Medical Agency. Guideline on bioanalytical method validation. 2011. Available at: http://www.ema.europa.eu/docs/en_GB/document_library/Scientific_guideline/2011/08/WC500109686.pdf. Accessed April, 2018.

10. Scientific Working Group for Forensic Toxicology. Scientific Working Group for Forensic Toxicology (SWGTOX) standard practices for method validation in forensic toxicology. J Anal Toxicol 2013;37(7):452–74.

11. Clinical and Laboratory Standards Institute (CLSI). Statistical quality control for quantitative measurement procedures: principles and definitions (C24). 4th edition. Wayne (PA): Clinical and Laboratory Standards Institute (CLSI); 2016.

12. Clinical and Laboratory Standards Institute (CLSI). Metrological traceability and its implementation (EP32). Wayne (PA): Clinical and Laboratory Standards Institute (CLSI); 2006.

13. Clinical and Laboratory Standards Institute (CLSI). Using proficiency testing and alternative assessment to improve medical laboratory quality (QMS24). 3rd edition. Wayne (PA): Clinical and Laboratory Standards Institute (CLSI); 2016.

14. College of American Pathologists (CAP). CAP accreditation program: chemistry and toxicology checklist. Northfield (IL): College of American Pathologists; 2016. Available at: http://www.cap.org/ShowProperty?nodePath=/UCMCon/Contribution%20Folders/DctmContent/education/OnlineCourseContent/2016/LAP-TLTMv2/checklists/cl-chm.pdf. Accessed April, 2018.

15. U.S Department of Health and Human Services, Food and Drug Administration, Center for Drug Evaluation and Research. Discussion paper on laboratory developed test, January 2017. Available at: https://www.fda.gov/downloads/medicaldevices/productsandmedicalprocedures/invitrodiagnostics/laboratorydevelopedtests/ucm536965.pdf. Accessed April, 2018.

Liquid Chromatography–Mass Spectrometry Education for Clinical Laboratory Scientists

Judith A. Stone, MT(ASCP), PhD, DABCC[a],*, Robert L. Fitzgerald, PhD, DABCC/T[b]

KEYWORDS

- Liquid-chromatography–tandem mass spectrometry • Training • Competency

KEY POINTS

- Quantitative liquid chromatography–tandem mass spectrometry (LC-MS/MS) as used in diagnostic laboratories is highly complex and requires a theoretic knowledge base and hands-on expertise by bench technologists, managers, and directors to insure acceptable quality and productivity.

- Training for quantitative LC-MS/MS is not included or is covered only briefly in programs for clinical laboratory scientists and may or may not be addressed in clinical chemistry fellowship and pathology residency training programs. As a consequence, training for this subspecialty takes place primarily on the job, within the diagnostic laboratories performing the testing.

- This article stratifies and lists the competencies required for bench personnel, research and development scientists who develop and validate methods, laboratory managers, and directors as an aid toward designing training curricula and assessing trainees and staff.

INTRODUCTION AND BACKGROUND

The world of quantitative diagnostic mass spectrometry (MS) is evolving toward automation and greater ease of use. For diagnostic laboratories, that means migration from manual procedures in esoteric testing sections of the laboratory to automated,

Disclosure Statement: J.A. Stone—travel expenses and honoraria as a short course instructor, Mass Spectrometry Applications to the Clinical Laboratory (MSACL), and consultant—Thermo-Fisher Scientific. R.L. Fitzgerald, travel expenses from MSACL, research support from Waters Corporation and Tecan Schweiz AG, travel expenses from the American Association for Clinical Chemistry.
[a] Toxicology/Mass Spectrometry Laboratory, University of California San Diego Health System, Center for Advanced Laboratory Medicine, Suite 150, Room 1314, 10300 Campus Point Drive, San Diego, CA 92121, USA; [b] Department of Pathology, University of California, San Diego, CA, USA
* Corresponding author.
E-mail address: jastone@ucsd.edu

high-throughput core laboratory sections. The holy grail of diagnostic MS automation is regulatory-compliant quantitative assays (eg, Food and Drug Administration approved or Conformité Européene [CE] mark) on a fully automated liquid chromatography (LC)–tandem mass spectrometry (MS/MS) instrument. Such a system would have ease of use similar to automated clinical chemistry analyzers—random-access workflow, minimal down-time, 24/7 service and support, and validated and ready-to-use reagents and calibrators supplied by the vendor. These systems would not require specialized end-user skills for operation and would have sampling and software that permit integration to track systems along with ASTM/HL7 interfaces to laboratory information systems.

A parallel goal is that no trade-off will have been made between ease of use and the impressive sensitivity, selectivity, and precision that are possible with LC-MS/MS. At this time, at least 1 vendor has made significant progress toward these goals and is poised to ship quantitative LC-MS/MS instruments designed for operation in highly automated diagnostic core laboratories.

To clarify terms, this article uses *diagnostic laboratory* to define settings in which the sole purpose of laboratory testing is to report results to the medical record for patient care in a regulated environment. Because MS is widely used in clinical research and clinical trials as well as diagnostic laboratories, *clinical MS* is defined as the much broader and less regulated practice encompassing all those activities, of which *diagnostic laboratory MS* is a smaller subset.

Why has quantitative LC-MS/MS remained, until now, a specialized practice, widely used in commercial diagnostic reference laboratories but not feasible in many hospital laboratories? Primary barriers for hospital laboratories are the expertise required to develop and validate procedures[1,2] and the challenging finances associated with large capital expenses for initial instrument purchases. In stark contrast, use of qualitative MS in the diagnostic microbiology laboratory has been rapidly adopted by most hospitals, transforming routine practice. The value proposition of matrix-assisted laser desorption/ionization (MALDI)-time of flight (TOF) in the microbiology laboratory is well justified based on reduced time to identification and decrease in reagent costs.[3,4] Because qualitative MALDI-TOF MS for diagnostic microbiology is becoming the norm, the technique is being integrated into training programs at all levels. The other rapidly developing field in diagnostic MS is imaging. The differences between training for imaging MS versus for quantitative LC-MS/MS are profound. Avoiding detail to address the 2 subspecialties in 1 article does both a disservice. Therefore, this article selectively addresses training for quantitative diagnostic LC-MS/MS, only 1 of the areas in which MS has become important in laboratory medicine.

If automated LC-MS/MS is widely implemented in core laboratories, then basic LC and MS/MS theory will become a standard feature in training curricula, as for spectrophotometry and electrophoresis. Will the need for personnel in diagnostic laboratories with specialized hands-on LC-MS/MS training disappear? An analogy can be made to typesetting—once a highly skilled, multifunctional profession that was made obsolete by revolutions in printing technology.[5] The premise of this article is that routine production with quantitative laboratory developed tests (LDTs) using stand-alone, open LC-MS/MS instruments will remain financially viable for some time in diagnostic laboratories. Therefore, the extensive training needed for such practice is described in detail.

Diagnostic laboratories that perform quantitative LC-MS/MS testing now have tremendous variance in their extent of automation, throughput, and test workload. The authors believe more useful descriptors than these to distinguish between current versus new MS testing paradigms are the site of assay development/validation and whether the LC-MS/MS system is open or closed. Open instruments can be used with assays from any source whereas closed systems are restricted to regulatory approved assays sold only by the instrument vendor. The traditional model of in-house test development/validation by the laboratory performing the assay on open LC-MS/MS systems are called LDT-open MS. The emerging system of regulatory-approved assays sold by in vitro diagnostic (IVD) companies for dedicated, closed systems are called IVD-closed MS. Laboratories performing Food and Drug Administration cleared or CE mark assays on open LC-MS/MS systems are considered in the LDT-open MS group.

This article describes training for LDT-open MS practice in sections defined first by function and secondarily by academic degree, licensure, and job title. Scientists with a bachelor of science degree and postbaccalaureate on-the-job training as well as physician-scientist laboratory directors with doctoral training in MS are successfully engaged in method development, validation, and troubleshooting for LDT-open MS laboratories. Because training and experience are so diverse in this field, desired competencies are focused on rather than academic qualifications and licensure.

TRAINING FOR BENCH PERSONNEL

Few training programs for diagnostic laboratory bench personnel in the United States include quantitative LC-MS/MS in their curriculum. An encouraging development is diagnostic MS coursework offered in a few academic clinical laboratory scientist (CLS) training programs, for example, Michigan State University and Virginia Commonwealth University. Short courses in quantitative diagnostic LDT-open MS are available online,[6] at scientific meetings,[7,8] and with a hands-on component[9] but are not included in the staff training budget of most diagnostic laboratories.

As a consequence, LDT-open MS diagnostic laboratories in North America expect to train all levels of personnel onsite. Although certification versus licensure has important distinctions, for the purposes of this article the terms are used interchangeably to indicate that a structured system for diagnostic laboratory personnel qualification has been defined by a regulatory body.

The bench tasks in an LDT-open MS laboratory are stratified by increasing skills and training:

1. Reagent and calibrator preparation
2. Sample preparation
3. Instrument operation (order of B and C may be reversed based on the level of automation)
4. Data analysis/review/reporting functions

Competencies recommended for these tasks are (assume appropriate active verbs as used in learning objections, such as *demonstrate*, *describe*, and *display*, precede all these listed functions) as follows.

Reagent Preparation

1. Correct use, cleaning, and storage of laboratory glassware for LC-MS/MS trace analysis
2. Competency with volumetric glassware, pH meters, analytical balances, positive displacement, air displacement and volumetric pipets
3. Best practices for handling of source materials (primary solvent containers, blank biological matrices, primary analytical standards [certified reference materials]) to avoid contamination from the environment or from improper containers

[e.g. phthalate plasticizers] or cross-contamination from mg/mL to pg/mL or analyte-free solutions
4. Measurement principles for solvents and water to achieve highly consistent solvent:water ratios of mobile phases and autosampler wash solutions
5. Laboratory safety (strong acids, bases, volatile organic solvents, and fire/explosion risk)
6. Lot, source material, and purity tracking, labeling for chemicals, solvents, and prepared reagent lots

Calibrator and Internal Standard Preparation

Consistent preparation of internal standards is important for the long-term stability of any quantitative LC-MS/MS assay and is more demanding of good laboratory technique than is simpler reagent preparation. In addition to the skills listed for reagent preparation, training and documented competency in the precise gravimetric and volumetric measurement of nonaqueous standard solutions (eg, stable isotope-labeled methanol stock solutions) is necessary.

The authors recommend a proficiency test of all new hires for pipetting and weighing performance. Competency testing should include gravimetrically assessed precision and accuracy with air displacement, positive displacement, and glass volumetric pipets for aqueous and nonaqueous liquids and gravimetric competency with National Institute of Standards and Technology–certified standard weights using an analytical balance.

Accurate calibrator preparation to within a ± 5% or 10% tolerance using certified primary stock solutions and validated blank biological matrices is a task that demands excellent laboratory technique. An alternative is custom calibrator preparation by a vendor, which can be surprisingly expensive. Calibrator preparation requires all the competencies listed for reagent and internal standard preparation as well as appropriate handling of expensive stock standards in volatile solvents and preventing cross-contamination from milligram per milliliter concentration stock standards to nanogram per milliliter or picogram per milliliter calibrator pools, laboratory consumables and pipets.

Sample Preparation

Manual sample preparation may persist in LDT-open MS laboratories as long as automated liquid handler (ALH) prices remain prohibitively high and batches of less than 100 samples are financially viable. Competencies for manual sample preparation include

1. Pipetting proficiency with air and positive displacement pipets with aqueous and nonaqueous solutions
2. Temperature and thermal equilibration effects on pipetting precision and accuracy
3. Best practices for avoiding cross-contamination between samples, reagents, internal standards, labware, and pipets
4. Calculations for and performing dilutions
5. Best practices for maintaining sample identification integrity with multiple transfers during extraction
6. Mitigation for nonspecific binding of measurands to surfaces (containers, caps, and so forth)
7. Plasticizer contamination from consumables (tubes, caps, parafilm sealant, and so forth)
8. Handling for alternate specimen types, such as oral fluid, meconium, and hair and tissue samples, for example, umbilical cord

9. Safe handling and disposal of acids, bases, organic solvents, body fluids, and tissues of human origin

Competency with extraction options other than dilution and protein precipitation may include but is not limited to

1. Solid-phase extraction media
2. Supported liquid extraction media
3. Liquid–liquid extraction
4. Protein precipitation filtration media
5. Phospholipid removal media
6. Tecan Immobilized Coating Extraction (Tecan Schweiz AG, Mannedorf, Switzerland)-coated AC Extraction Plate
7. Trypsin digestion for protein analyses
8. Glucuronide hydrolysis of urine samples
9. Stable Isotope Standards and Capture by Anti-Peptide Antibodies workflows for protein and peptide measurands

Use of ALH for LC-MS/MS sample preparation can deliver major advances in productivity. ALH programming is complex, however, and requires instrument-specific software training. Proficiency at programming ALH may have less relation to level of formal education and be more closely associated with a talent for process improvement, compulsive attention to detail, tolerance of excessive iteration for optimizing liquid handling steps, and basic programming capabilities. Recommended competencies for programmers/key operators of ALH include

1. Software version control, backup, and documentation best practices
2. Liquid handling basic principles for aqueous and nonaqueous fluids
3. Basic robotics programming—principles covered in vendor training courses, for example
4. Best practices for ALH script or program validation and documentation
5. Completion of an ALH vendor's training course or comparable in-house training with assessment

In contrast, operators of ALH for production who do not program and use only validated pipetting/extraction methods may not require extensive training. Safety training to prevent injury from or damage to robotic arms or pipetting channels is a priority.

The most useful competencies may be for recovery from human error, such as

1. Misplaced labware
2. Misplaced carriers
3. Misplaced reagents and samples
4. Selecting the wrong script
5. Software-hardware communication errors
6. Shortages of tips, plates, reagents

Liquid Chromatography–Tandem Mass Spectrometry Instrument Operation, Maintenance, and Troubleshooting

Daily LC-MS/MS maintenance and routine batch submission for LDT-open MS systems is done in some laboratories by unlicensed personnel, with limited LC-MS/MS training. This can work well as long as there are no problems. Review of LC-MS/MS system suitability test (SST) results, MS/MS component cleaning and replacement, LC plumbing, and troubleshooting, however, requires not only hands-on experience but also knowledge of LC and MS/MS theory.

One approach is to stratify instrument operators on the premise that an 80:20 rule applies. This assumes that 80% of batches are problem-free so routine operators need less expertise. With good procedures in place for recognition and referral of problems, the 20% of problematic runs can be referred to a subset of troubleshooting personnel with higher-level LC-MS/MS competency. In smaller laboratories, the expertise needed for complex troubleshooting overlaps with that for method development; hence, the same person may fulfill both job functions.

Basic operator competencies:

1. Daily check, replacing of instrument fluids, liquid waste disposal
2. Daily check, recording of instrument parameters—gas pressures and supplies, vacuum pressures
3. Daily check of thresholds for replacing chromatography consumables
4. Basic computer maintenance
5. Manual install of computer operating system updates, antivirus updates (if not scheduled)
6. Remove/clean/reinstall atmospheric pressure source components (eg, curtain plate, cone, or skimmer)
7. Run SST

Troubleshooting competencies—the LC is the source of most problems. This list, therefore, emphasizes LC skills[10] and the terms, *recognize*, *solve*, and *develop*, are the active verbs that should precede many of these learning objectives:

1. Stationary/mobile-phase differences between reverse-phase and hydrophilic interaction liquid chromatography
2. Effects on LC back pressures of column architecture, mobile-phase composition, flow rate, temperature:
   a. LC stationary-phase particle size
   b. LC column dimensions
3. Problems caused by excess LC extracolumn dead volume
4. Problems caused by aged LC components
5. Rules for composition of injection matrix
6. Sources of column overload (volume overload, mismatch of injection solvent and mobile-phase conditions, and mass overload)
7. LC pressure traces to find leaks, overpressure, and aged LC pump check valves
8. SST, maintenance calendar annotation, and postcolumn infusion to distinguish between human error, sample preparation, and LC or MS/MS instrument failure
9. Isolate LC segments with overpressure or obscure leaks.
10. Change LC pump check valves, plunger seals, and plungers; dispel air from the LC pump head.
11. Change autosampler needle, needle seal/seat, sample loops, and syringes, and dispel airlocks.
12. Problems of no baseline/no peaks/shifted retention times/abnormal baseline/abnormal peak shape
13. Perform MS/MS detector voltage optimization test
14. Change MS/MS source components
15. Problems with failing vacuum systems
16. Ballast and change oil for foreline (roughing) vacuum pumps.
17. Investigate need for MS/MS interface cleaning.
18. Vent and pump down the MS/MS.
19. Exchange used for cleaned/new MS/MS interface components (ion guides).

20. Perform mass resolution and calibration, evaluate reports.
21. Use of qualitative data review to compare and contrast shifts and trends in signal-to-noise ratio, peak shape, and retention time

Quantitative Liquid Chromatography–Tandem Mass Spectrometry Data Review and Reporting

The availability of sophisticated automation software for data review (eg, Indigo ASCENT [BioAutomation, Carmel, Indiana], MultiQuant [SCIEX, Framingham, MA], and Skyline [MacCoss Lab Software, University of Washington, Seattle, WA]) with options for "review by exception" has changed expectations for this component of the LDT-open MS workflow.[11–14] Competencies necessary for manual data review are listed, with the expectation that similar expertise is required for review by exception but with large improvements in throughput due to the limited number of chromatograms that require review when auto-verification rules are applied. The learning objective terms preceding many of these items should be *recognize deviation*, *find the source of the problem*, and *apply corrective action for*.

1. Abnormal peak shape, detector saturation, unacceptably low signal-to-noise ratio, dwell time errors
2. Peak shape degradation for 1 versus all samples in a batch
3. Trends/shifts in LC-MS/MS metadata, for example, ion ratios, internal standard peak areas
4. Retention time (Rt), relative retention time flagging, variance, trends, shifts, and acceptable versus unacceptable deviations
5. Blank sample acceptance criteria and review for carryover from high to low concentration samples
6. Drug and hormone metabolite abnormalities
7. Review of calibration curve parameter and acceptance criteria
8. Quality control (QC) failures
9. Referral criteria for secondary review, sample rejection, reinjection, repeat extraction, dilution, and customized report comments
10. Maintenance of batch records

TRAINING FOR METHOD VALIDATION AND DEVELOPMENT

The authors are not aware of any academic training specific for diagnostic quantitative LC-MS/MS method development and validation. Clinical chemistry fellowships and short courses (American Society for Mass Spectrometry (ASMS) and Mass Spectrometry: Applications to the Clinical Laboratory (MSACL)) are the best training resources to the authors' knowledge.[7,8] The most effective training for this highly complex task is exposure in a diagnostic laboratory to a mentor with experience and expertise in both LDT-open MS and laboratory medicine.

The skills and experience needed to implement robust methods for production are not well characterized. What do we mean by *robust* and *production*? Production is defined as daily reporting of results from validated LDT-open MS quantitative assays in a regulated diagnostic laboratory. Robust is less easy to characterize. Differences of note between less regulated research MS assays and the performance of and practice necessary for production assays that can be described as robust include

1. Reliability (low rate of batch failures) and better precision (eg, CVs <10%)
2. Less than or equal to 15% between sample variance in matrix effect after correction for internal standard response

3. Faster turnaround times with low exception rates
4. Extensive validation (eg, Clinical & Laboratory Standards Institute (CLSI) C62-A document and other CLSI guidance)
5. Routine tracking of SST results and MS/MS metadata with validated action limits
6. Routine tracking of reagent, solvent, chemical, internal standard, calibrator, and consumable lots with lot to lot validation testing
7. QC schema, action limits, and review consistent with regulatory requirements
8. As available, uninterrupted chain of traceability to standard reference materials
9. Testing can be performed by CLS level personnel

The following competencies are proposed for robust method development/validation personnel:

1. All skills listed previously for materials preparation, sample preparation, instrument operation, troubleshooting, and data review
2. Writing development and validation plans
3. Developing an MS/MS method
   a. Selecting, optimizing MRMs, dwell times, and grouping/timing of Multiple Reaction monitoring precursor/product ion pairs for optimal points/peak
   b. Optimizing source parameters
      i. Using design of experiments for source optimization
   c. Characterizing ionization based on mobile-phase composition, positive/negative mode
4. Screening and selecting LC columns, guard columns, inline filters, and mobile phases
   a. High-throughput screening of stationary phases, column dimensions, and particle types with automation
5. Minimizing LC dead volume
6. Developing an LC gradient, screening gradients
   a. High-throughput screening of solvents/gradients with automation—see also "4".
   b. 2-D LC
   c. High-temperature LC
   d. Online solid phase extraction
   e. LC multiplexing
7. Defining boundaries for injection solution solvent, pH composition, and injection volume
8. Evaluating analyte chemistry and desired lower limit of quantitation to select sample preparation options
9. Knowledge of common sample preparation methods for LDT-open MS, options to concentrate analytes while depleting matrix
10. Quantifying extraction precision, recovery, and matrix effect
    a. Optimizing extraction, LC, and MS/MS to minimize matrix effect variance
    b. Screening for nonspecific binding, solubility problems
11. Use of postcolumn infusion to optimize LC gradients and sample preparation and reduce between-sample variance in matrix effect
12. Use of single-source native matrix samples early in development
13. Defining the analytical measurement range, validating precision at the lower limit of quantitation
14. Designing calibration strategies and materials
15. Selection of QC materials and concentrations

16. Concepts of method robustness, process optimization, minimizing liquid transfers, and optimizing extraction containers
17. Prevalidation studies
18. Fit for purpose validation of methods and compliance with regulatory guidance
19. Writing validation reports
20. Writing Standard operating procedure (SOPs), training production personnel
21. Transitioning methods to production

TRAINING TO MANAGE PRODUCTION AND QUALITY

Supervisors and managers with diagnostic laboratory but no MS experience may find it challenging to adapt to oversight of LDT-open MS laboratories. The advantage of LC-MS/MS technology is that many more options exist to assess and control quality than with less complex measurement techniques. Every result from an LC-MS/MS system has a wealth of instrument metadata that can be used to evaluate the acceptability of the analysis. Although less accessible, in diagnostic laboratories there should also be noninstrument information documented for each result (lot and source material validation, QC and sample preparation history, analyst competency, batch records, instrument SST, and service records). The difficulty is that most open source data management and automation solutions for creating, storing, queries of, and useful presentation for LDT-open MS big data were developed for proteomics research and only recently have been applied in diagnostic laboratories.[14-17] The authors know of no formal training for, but believe that managers should become familiar with and may want to implement, the solutions and best practices recommended:

1. Centralized (secure server) storage of all LC-MS/MS raw data with automated backup
2. Automated tracking of SST results with exception flagging, notification, and remote review capability
3. Software to mine archived LC-MS/MS metadata for between batch, short-term, and longer-term monitoring to forecast instrument/batch failure and track metrics to improve method robustness
4. Database storage, tracking, and queries for information NOT stored in laboratory information or QC software systems, such as
   a. Lots in use for chromatography consumables
   b. Lots in use and certificates of analysis for primary standards
   c. Lots in use for water, chemicals, solvents and prepared reagents, calibrators, and lot-to-lot validations
   d. Instrument maintenance and service records
   e. Batch records
   f. LC- MS/MS, ALH method edits, version control, and SOP document control
   g. Autoverification rules validation and version control

TRAINING FOR INSTRUMENT SELECTION, TEST MENU, AND CLINICAL OVERSIGHT BY LABORATORY DIRECTORS

Formal training for directors of LDT-open MS laboratories takes place in some but not all clinical postdoctoral fellowship and laboratory physician (clinical pathology and medical biochemistry) residency programs. The degree to which doctoral scientists and physicians engage in learning the technical and informatics competencies described in this article for LDT-open MS varies with the training program and the trainee. Board certification examinations are increasingly likely to include questions about LC and MS/MS theory and practice. The authors recommend the following competencies specifically for training directors of LDT-open MS laboratory sections. They also may be useful for generalist laboratory directors who should be aware of the challenges to using MS technology in the diagnostic laboratory and need to assess the qualifications of candidates to direct LDT-open MS laboratory sections.

1. Basics of quadrupole and hybrid MS/MS theory and function
2. Differences between triple quadrupole, time of flight, and (Orbitrap mass analyzer, Waltham, MA) for quantitation
3. Compromises between ideal function and routine performance of LDT-open MS and IVD-closed MS production instruments in diagnostic laboratories
4. Basics of LC theory, practice, optimization, and limitations when used with MS/MS for quantitation
5. Compare and contrast sample preparation methods for quality, cost, and productivity (less sample cleanup may translate to more instrument down time)
6. Basic principles of LDT-open MS method development, validation, implementation, and quality management in production as appropriate for job function
7. Selection of and implementing training, assessing initial competency, and continuing performance for personnel who will perform LDT-open MS bench testing, method development and validation, quality management, and production oversight
8. Leadership, collaboration, or delegation to implement evolving informatics solutions for LDT-open MS automation and quality management
9. Strategies for increasing LC-MS/MS throughput and selectivity (LC multiplexing, MS/MS multiplexing, and developing technologies [eg, ion mobility])
10. Writing return on investment and request for proposal/tender documents for instrument purchase
11. Communicating the value of MS testing to clinicians and recruiting clinician support for MS instrument purchase
12. Selecting team members for instrument purchase due diligence
13. Ranking vendors and quotations, negotiating for instrument purchase, service contracts, and training and application support
14. Engagement with clinicians, laboratory, finance, and regulatory administrators to assess LDT-open MS versus IVD-closed MS testing demand, laboratory budgets, test reimbursement, and constructing and modifying LDT-open MS test menus

SUMMARY

A menu of competencies is proposed in some detail for personnel working in LDT-open MS diagnostic laboratories. The goal is that online training resources, short courses, and clinical chemistry postdoctoral fellowship and residency training programs can use and further develop these guidelines to the benefit of their trainees.

REFERENCES

1. Vogeser M. Mass Spectrometry in the clinical laboratory—challenges for quality assurance. Spectroscopy 2015;13:14–9.
2. Education and expense: the barriers to mass spectrometry in clinical laboratories? Technology networks. 2015. Available at: https://www.technologynetworks.com/analysis/news/education-and-expense-the-barriers-to-mass-spectrometry-in-clinical-laboratories-193157. Accessed May 2, 2018.
3. Paxton A. MALDI in microbiology: set to stun? CAP Today 2015.

4. Tan KE, Ellis BC, Lee R, et al. Prospective evaluation of a matrix-assisted laser desorption ionization-time of flight mass spectrometry system in a hospital clinical microbiology laboratory for identification of bacteria and yeasts: a bench-by-bench study for assessing the impact on time to identification and cost-effectiveness. J Clin Microbiol 2012;50:3301–8.
5. Romano F. The day the typesetting industry died. WhatTheyThink, Market Intelligence for Printing and Publishing; 2011. Available at: http://whattheythink.com/articles/55522-day-typesetting-industry-died/. Accessed May 2, 2018.
6. American Association for Clinical Chemistry online certificate programs, Introductory Liquid Chromatography Mass Spectrometry for the Clinical Laboratory and LC-MS/MS Troubleshooting for the Clinical Laboratory. Available at: https://www.aacc.org/education-and-career/online-certificate-programs/laboratory-technology. Accessed May 2, 2018.
7. Mass Spectrometry Applications to the Clinical Laboratory (MSACL) Short Courses at United States and European meetings. Available at: https://www.msacl.org/index.php?header=MSACL_2018_US&tab=Details&subtab=Short_Courses. Accessed May 2, 2018.
8. American Society for Mass Spectrometry (ASMS) Annual Meeting Short Courses, 02 Clinical Diagnostics: Innovation, Validation, Implementation and Operation by Mass Spectrometry. Available at: http://www.asms.org/docs/default-source/conference-short-course-descriptions/02-clinical-diagnostic-testing.pdf?sfvrsn=2. Accessed May 2, 2018.
9. Ritchie J, Botelho J, Vesper H. Performing clinical testing using mass spectrometry – hands-on training. Emory University/CDC Joint Center for Mass Spectrometry and Advanced Technology. Available at: https://www.msacl.org/documents/hands-on-training/20180326_HandsOn_ClinicalMS_Brochure.pdf. Accessed May 2, 2018.
10. Stoll DR. Resources for lc practitioners in 2017: what's on your bookshelf and in your web browser? LCGC 2017;35:854–61.
11. Dickerson J, Mathias P. Making a case for automated data review. Washington, DC: Clin Lab News; 2016.
12. Alexander K, Terrell AR. Automated review of mass spectrometry results can we achieve autoverification? Clin Lab News; 2015.
13. Henderson CM, Shulman NJ, MacLean B, et al. Skyline performs as well as vendor software in the quantitative analysis of serum 25-hydroxy vitamin D and vitamin D binding globulin. Clin Chem 2018;64:408–10.
14. Panorama: repository software for targeted mass spectrometry assays from skyline. Available at: https://panoramaweb.org/project/home/begin.view? Accessed April 2, 2018.
15. Zabell A, Stone JA, Julian RK. Using big data for LC-MS/MS quality analysis. Washington, DC: Clin Lab News; 2017.
16. Bittremieux W, Willems H, Keighterman P, et al. iMonDB: mass spectrometry quality control through instrument monitoring. J Proteome Res 2015;14:2360–6.
17. Dogu E, Mohammad-Taheri S, Abbatiello SE, et al. MSstatsQC: longitudinal system suitability monitoring and quality control for targeted proteomic experiments. Mol Cell Proteomics 2017;16:1335–47.

Special Considerations for Liquid Chromatography–Tandem Mass Spectrometry Method Development

Brian A. Rappold, PhD

KEYWORDS

- Method development • Liquid chromatography • Mass spectrometry • Endogenous
- Internal standards • Validation

KEY POINTS

- Optimization of liquid chromatography–tandem mass spectrometry methods during development is iterative through the developmental pipeline.
- Isotopically labeled internal standards provide near perfect surrogates for endogenous analytes when testing true human matrices.
- Modulation of chromatographic separations can elucidate nonspecificity of detection and should be used in method development.
- Aspects of method development that are outside commonplace evaluations include assessments of stoichiometry in pathologic states for derivatized workflows, area ratio monitoring for precision evaluations, and assessment of multiple sources of calibration material.

Method development for liquid chromatography–tandem mass spectrometry (LC-MS/MS) assays involves numerous components, including the varieties of sample preparation and LC as well as the advantages and limitations of MS. It is not uncommon that a simplistic view is provided with regard to method development, particularly in publications, which undervalues the complexity of method development. For example, sample preparation is generally divided into 4 classes, all of which may be used in the same workflow, those being protein precipitation (or simple dilution), liquid-liquid extraction, solid-phase extraction, and analyte modification (eg, derivatization or proteolysis). Yet within each of those procedures is a host of possibilities and variables: solid-phase extraction might use ion exchange, hydrophobic or hydrophilic mechanisms, or a combination. And each mechanism might use a variety of solvents, stationary phase ligands, stationary phase masses, wash steps, stationary phase-drying steps, elution steps, and evaporation/reconstitution steps, with each iteration possibly playing an essential role in the viability of the assay to be applied to the analysis of human specimens for diagnostic purposes. The landscape for method development is extensive.

Disclosure: The author has no commercial or financial interests in the article.
Mass Spectrometry Laboratory Corporation of America, 1904 TW Alexander Drive, Durham, NC 27703, USA
E-mail address: rappolb@labcorp.com

Unfortunately, many of the details regarding method development are not included in descriptions found in most journals. Seemingly, method development occurs with only a plurality of positive outcomes. Articles often report final results for method development, not the actual method development itself. Take for example, a recent reference method procedure for amyloid beta 1 to 42, which uses ion exchange solid-phase extraction.[1] The investigators note adding additional washes to a previously published procedure, including a 4% aqueous phosphoric acid wash and increasing elution volumes. It is unclear what benefit a strong acid wash and changes in elution volume yielded, and perhaps more importantly, how those modifications were scientifically determined to be appropriate. That is not to say that the assay is unsuitable, but it does point out the absence of a description of method development. Rather, it includes a description of the final method. This might be because many experimental results in method development are negative and there is a bias toward not publishing negative outcomes.[2]

MASS SPECTROMETRY

Determination of MS parameters is generally the first step in method development. Identification of initial parameters, such as precursor ions, product ions, and source conditions must be established before further assay interrogation. Simply, data from chromatographic and sample preparation are fallible when detection is not performed in a consistent and high-quality manner. Many assays use multiple precursor-product transitions of a single analyte in the assessment of ion ratios to provide additional confidence in results. At the onset of development, the purity of a peak in human specimens (selectivity) has not been determined. As such, all available transitions should be maintained until such point that a precursor/production pair can be determined to be useful as a quantitative ion, a qualifying ion, or is excluded as being susceptible to interferences. The choice of removing a transition in method development should be entirely driven by specificity of analysis; dose-response functions for a particular ion transition can be modulated by ionization cross-section, dissociation efficiency, sample preparation, sample volume used and load of the sample in to the instrument. Given the ability of current-day MSs to scan quickly across multiple transitions, development of assays should move forward with all available possibilities until data definitively prove the quality of a particular MS/MS transition.

Notably, however, there are certain transitions that must be used with care.[3,4] When using MS/MS transitions that are either ubiquitous or facile, ensuring reproducibility and specificity in many authentic human specimens should be extensively evaluated in prevalidation and well proven in validation.

Reproducibility of a particular transition is quickly assessed by an evaluation of analyte to internal standard peak area ratios in early method development. In mass spectrometric assays with isotopically labeled internal standards (IS), it is assumed that most analytical variation is normalized by the IS. Inaccuracy should then be attributable only to the aliquoting of sample and the addition of IS. In practice, however, there may be some inaccuracy in the detection of compounds related to in-source variation or dissociation differences. **Table 1** shows exemplar data from the performance of this experiment for oxycodone using 2 transitions for the analyte and 2 transitions for the internal standard. Here, the analyte and internal standard are aliquoted to a single vial in neat solvent at a concentration intended to yield a moderate response in the mass spectrometer (high enough to provide confidence in the signal, low enough to avoid source and detector nonlinearity). The solution is injected in replicates (20 in this example) to determine the imprecision of analyte peak area to

Table 1		
Precision of analyte/IS transitions in development		
	Oxycodone 1	**Oxycodone 2**
Analyte transition	316.2 → 256.1	316.2 → 187.1
IS transition	319.2 → 259.1	319.2 → 190.1
	Area Ratio, Oxycodone 1	**Area Ratio, Oxycodone 2**
Low sample 1	0.192	0.178
Low sample 2	0.177	0.214
Low sample 3	0.203	0.197
Low sample 4	0.204	0.24
Low sample 5	0.204	0.19
Low sample 6	0.198	0.217
Low sample 7	0.181	0.225
Low sample 8	0.185	0.227
Low sample 9	0.196	0.202
Low sample 10	0.182	0.202
Low sample 11	0.202	0.218
Low sample 12	0.188	0.191
Low sample 13	0.204	0.193
Low sample 14	0.198	0.228
Low sample 15	0.183	0.213
Low sample 16	0.202	0.195
Low sample 17	0.182	0.234
Low sample 18	0.191	0.22
Low sample 19	0.206	0.208
Low sample 20	0.192	0.198
Mean	0.1935	0.2095
SD	0.009417229	0.016687531
CV	4.87%	7.97%

Assessment of analyte-to-IS area ratios for determination of transition precision in method development. A single mixed sample injected 20 times indicates a higher imprecision for the Oxycodone 2 transition, providing a preference for Oxycodone 1 in quantification.

internal standard peak area ratios. Observing that the oxycodone 1 transition is notably better than oxycodone 2 transition (coefficient of variation (CV's) of 4.87% and 7.97%) indicates a preference for the oxycodone 1 transition to be used in quantitation for further development. It also may be the method developer's intention to achieve lower precision values, indicating the need to address the variation in the first transition.

Another key consideration is that the ion source conditions established in preliminary evaluations may not be optimal for the final assay. Many initial determinations of MS parameters are performed at a low flow infusion of the compound(s) of interest in a neat solution. This solution will certainly differ from the final eluent conditions of the analyte(s) following preparation and LC. Optimization of parameters in the source of the mass spectrometer, including temperature, declustering potential, gas flows, and ionization voltage, should be performed as iterative steps during the process of development and revisited when a relevant parameter becomes a variable.[5,6]

It should be noted here that in development of an LC-MS/MS assay, there are but 2 possible components that might be used to yield higher response functions. The first would be in the volume of sample used in processing. If unacceptable signal is observed at 100 μL of sample extracted, using 300 μL in sample preparation should theoretically triple the response produced, given the same final volume (assuming all other variables in the LC-MS/MS process are unaffected by sample volume). Alternatively, injecting 3-fold more sample onto the LC column should also yield a theoretic 3-fold increase (note that this is not always true for a variety of reasons, but that does not detract from the point being made here).[7]

Care should be taken in rationalizing the use of higher sample volume to achieve lower limits of measurement. In certain assays, such as those evaluating neonates, limitations in available blood volume may be prohibitive in discrete veins. Operationally, requesting large volumes of sample from certain patient populations can be difficult.

The second is in the source of the mass spectrometer, in which ion yield is dependent on a number of controllable factors. Improving ionization cross-section, in contrast to sample volume, presents a fairly painless mechanism to achieve lower limits of detection. Both controlled variables, such as temperature and gas flow, as well as uncontrolled variables, such as cleanliness of ion optics or electrodes, affect the generation and yield of ions from the mass spectrometer's source. The experimental space for increasing ion yields also encompasses solvent chemistry, such as solution pH, mobile phase's constituents, and additives.[8,9] Experimental paradigms to evaluate ionization differences has been described in detail elsewhere.[10] Also for consideration is the manufacturing source of solvents, as there may be significant differences in the response on analytes based on the manufacturer of a "pure" solvent.[11,12] Careful interpretation of the data is critical to the decision-making process, as not all changes may exhibit a consistent effect.[13]

LIQUID CHROMATOGRAPHY DEVELOPMENT

Resolution of compounds in a time dimension is critical to the claimed selectivity of mass spectrometric analysis in diagnostics. Isobaric species, or molecules that are observed in the same mass transitions as a compound of interest, are common features, particularly for classes of biomarkers with conserved chemical structures (ie, steroids). Analytically, these might be a result of isomers, isotopes, or derived from interactions in the mass spectrometer's source.[14] In the clinical setting, a host of interfering signals may be observed due to uncommon molecules produced in vivo as a function of disease, lifestyle, diet, a medication, polypharmacy, or other untraceable preanalytical confounders. Given the variety of the human population that might be tested and a maximal capacity of ion generation, MS alone is incapable of addressing the milieu of possible interfering species, hence the need for LC and sample preparation.

Given the absence of chromatographic theory described in publications for diagnostic assays, it is recommended that method development focuses on empirical processes, using experience and intuition in interpreting results. Relevant experimental outcomes, such as "is the compound retained," are fundamental questions that should be answered in development. As it relates to diagnostic testing, chromatographic methods must include screening against isobaric species, identification of ionization-modifying regions of a chromatogram, and determining specificity in authentic specimens.

Possibly interfering compounds in biological fluids may be difficult to predict when measured by MS. However, some effort should be applied in the development of a new assay to evaluate the potential appearance of such species. One route for exploring possible isobars is related to searching for compounds with the same pseudomolecular ion or even common types of ions generated.[15] The freely obtainable information found in the supplemental data of the referenced article yields a variety of substances that, given commercial availability, should be purchased and used in chromatographic development if reasonable concern exists that such a compound could present as an interferent in analysis. Certain compounds may not be an issue; an isobaric species for 1,25 dihydroxyvitamin D ($C_{27}H_{44}O_3$, $[M+H]^+ = 417.3$) may be $C_2H_{40}O_{22}$ (predicted $[M+H]^+ = 417.2$), as the 2 molecules would be within unit resolution in the first stage of quadrupole mass analysis, but that molecule would not be of concern, as it would be an unlikely candidate for protonation as well as unlikely to exist in nature.

Certain endogenous substances are known to influence the ionization of analytes. The magnitude of the effect is dependent on a number of factors related to the preparative, chromatographic, and ionization modes and platforms. It is generally accepted that phospholipids and phthalates disrupt normal ionization in electrospray MS.[16] In blood-based matrices collected under normal processes, these compound classes are ubiquitous and, at times, substantially concentrated. Luckily, these species are observable in the mass spectrometer, allowing for the identification of possible elution regions where, in the absence of sample preparation intended to remove such compounds, confidence in precise detection is minimized.[17] Similar to the addition of known isobaric species when evaluating chromatographic systems, inclusion of the transitions for analytes that are known to present issues in analysis is highly recommended. For example, development of methylmalonic acid in serum measured the most abundant lysolipid and phospholipid species during chromatographic screening to ensure that co-elution, and thus ion suppression, would not be a pervasive issue.[18]

As chromatographic method development progresses and confidence builds in the reliability of the method, an evaluation of human specimens must be performed. This should occur as early in method development as possible to identify possible errors that will need to be addressed in other phases of method development. Such errors might include poor response of the analyte at the intended lower limit of measurement interval in authentic samples (recovery in neat solutions is only a proxy for retention time, peak shape, and resolution) or the identification of interfering peaks. A simple experiment to determine peak authenticity is to increase resolution in the chromatographic separation through increasing the retention of the compound. In isocratic separations, this is performed by lowering the percentage of the eluotropic content in the mobile phase and increasing the run. A gradient separation's time must be extended such that the peak and its possible interferences exhibit increased resolution (decreased change in eluotropic content over time). Samples are injected on the method intended for use from development and reinjected on the extended method. Data review can be performed by assessment of the analyte-to-IS area ratio, ion ratios, or simply peak counting.

In the analysis of norbuprenorphine, it was determined that all transitions suffer an interferent peak by changes in the transition ratios. The sample shown in **Fig. 1** was originally assayed using a methanol water linear gradient with the column at 50°C (**Fig. 1A**). Peaks for all transitions were consistent in shape and retention time, although transition ratios were outside of expected values. Thus, the gradient time was tripled with the same terminal percent organic (reduced slope of percent organic change over time) and the sample reinjected. Baseline resolution of norbuprenorphine and the unknown metabolite is achieved indicating a lack of specificity in analysis.

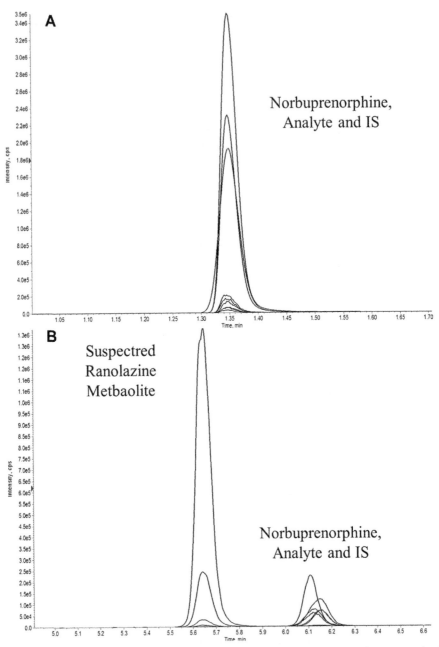

Fig. 1. Extended gradient separation: LC-MS/MS analysis of norbuprenorphine in method development. Screening of the human matrix indicated an unresolved peak identified only by transition ratio assessments. The water:methanol gradient time was extended from 2.5 to 7.5 minutes and the samples re-assayed. (*A*) The short gradient. (*B*) Baseline resolved peaks representing the interferent (5.6 minutes), norbuprenorphine's internal standard (6.12 minutes), and norbuprenorphine (6.15 minutes).

SAMPLE PREPARATION

Decision making related to which sample preparation technique to apply should be driven by the level of complexity required. The use of simple dilution is preferred over more convoluted approaches unless data indicate that simple dilution is not an appropriate path to assay validity. Any scheme that removes the opportunity for error in analysis should be implemented, including automation.[19] Simplification of sample handling and removing transfer steps should reduce the possibilities of cross-contamination, lost specimens, or other errors.

To evaluate various modalities of sample preparation, experiments should not be based primarily on the recovery of analyte from neat solutions, but should also monitor recovery of the analyte(s) and internal standard(s) from human specimens. This process of adding internal standard, however, deserves some scrutiny. Analytes may have binding partners (specific or nonspecific) and in some cases with high affinity.[20] If the internal standard is added to sample, briefly mixed, and immediately extracted, equilibrium of the internal standard with the sample's binding proteins may not have occurred. This could result in underrecovery of the analyte in relation to the internal standard, and thus a lower reported concentration. Evaluation of equivalent recovery could be assessed by sequential sampling and immediate extraction of samples that have been spiked with the internal standard and allowed to come to equilibrium. Within the same sample, a ratio of the analyte and internal standard should be precise in the absence of binding-associated recovery issues in a similar data output to **Table 1**.

Also of concern is loss of analyte due to the adsorption onto the surfaces of pipette tips and or containers for samples during handling. This has been previously reported for molecules such as the 11-Nor-9-carboxy- tetrahydrocannabinol, a metabolite of tetrahydrocannabinol.[21] Broadly, evaluations of adsorptive losses are not discussed in method development publications, although a protocol has been presented previously.[22,23]

Specific sample preparation techniques have been evaluated in detail.[24] Additionally, solid-phase extraction,[25] protein precipitation,[26,27] and online extraction[28] are possible tools in method development. The predominant concerns for sample preparation are related to the absolute recovery or yield of analyte from the process, as well as matrix effects.[29–31] The ability to identify experimentally the step in the process yielding unexpected signal losses (either from recovery or ionization suppression) is key to quality method development.

An aspect to sample preparation using derivatization of compounds to provide some requisite performance characteristic is not uncommon in LC-MS/MS workflows. Some benefits might include appropriate chromatographic retention in familiar LC modalities (as in derivatization of highly polar compounds to achieve reverse-phase retention),[32] increases in response functions for poorly ionized analytes,[33] or reducing data complexity through use of certain "tagging" strategies.[34] Undisclosed in most method development publications, however, is an evaluation of stoichiometry in the pathologic samples exhibiting perturbed biological functions.

Many biomarkers are assessed for their upregulation in relationship to a disorder. However, a biomarker may not be the only elevated species in a pathologic state, but just the one that provides the highest degree of clinical sensitivity and specificity for a particular disorder. When considering stoichiometry, fortification of solely the biomarker into human matrix as an evaluation of complete conversion is inappropriate. That approach assumes that only the biomarker of interest consumes the derivatization reagent and does not react with any other available species, especially those that are in high abundance as a function of altered metabolism or underlying disease.

INTERNAL STANDARDS

The choice of IS is often simplified to the availability of a material from commercial vendors. Although custom synthesis is possible, deployment of an assay may be delayed due to cost or reliability of such synthesis. Regardless of origin, it could be claimed that an isotopically labeled internal standard is perhaps the distinguishing feature of MS/MS detection; without it, MS/MS suffers the same, if not more, of the limitations of other technologies related to matrix effects and variability in recovery.

Briefly, ISs should be labeled at least 3 mass units above the nominal mass of the analyte, although in certain instances a higher degree of labeling is necessary to prevent contribution from naturally occurring analyte isotopes to the signal of the internal standard. Compounds that contain atoms with a variety of isotopes, such as chlorine, should be assessed for such contribution with care. When assessing particularly large molecules, the possible isotopic contributions from high concentrations of analyte should be evaluated for addition to IS signal. An assessment of isotopic contribution should take into account the relative signal change in the IS and its effect on both analytical performance (ie, addition to the IS at 3% contribution may be meaningless in context of the assay's inaccuracy), as well as clinical performance (ie, a high level of analyte induces a negative bias in the reported concentration, but a positive result is sufficient for the assay's intended use).[35] Additionally, ISs should be reviewed for contribution to analyte signal from either manufacturing impurities (incomplete isotopic incorporation) or, in the case of deuterated compounds, hydrogen-deuterium exchange. Hydrogen-deuterium exchange can occur either in solution or in the source of the mass spectrometer.[36]

As a tool for method development, the internal standard should mirror the extraction, chromatographic, and mass spectrometric characteristics of the analyte. This analogous performance is informative, particularly for the assessment of endogenous compounds. The use of an isotopically labeled version of the molecule may act as a surrogate when the authentic matrix contains the analyte of interest.[1] As such, all available MS/MS transitions for the IS should be monitored during all prevalidation experiments to mimic those of analyte as well as to determine reliability of those IS transitions. Secondary, or qualifying, transitions should be used to assess IS peak purity; there should be no belief that an IS peak is pure just because it has a non-natural distribution of isotopes.

A direct surrogate approach can be used for many of the experiments in method development by fortifying the IS in place of the analyte wherever data are complicated by the possibility of nonselectivity, questionable ionization consistency, or uncertain experimental outcomes (ie, proteolysis screening conditions where no response may be due poor sample preparation, poor enzyme kinetics, degradation, or matrix effects).[37] Additionally, the internal standard can be used as the direct observation of performance in chromatographic method development, as the use of real human specimens early in that paradigm is critical to efficient new assay maturation. For example, spiking of internal standard into human matrix extracts and neat solution can be highly informative for ion suppression or enhancement as well as for preliminary specificity evaluations while screening various chromatographic modalities. The difference between response of the IS in human matrix versus neat solution can indicate matrix effects. Chromatographic development with both the analyte and the internal standard in true matrix can reveal selectivity issues if retention times and peak widths do not align between the 2 compound types.

Despite all the benefits offered by an isotopically labeled IS, there is some concern related to a lack of co-elution between an analyte and its IS, particularly if the IS includes deuterium as the label.[38,39] The differences between hydrogen and deuterium are significant enough that the analyte and the internal standard elute in different regions of the chromatogram possibly subject the 2 compounds to distinct ionization efficiencies, either by solvent composition or co-eluting materials. Indeed, assays using deuterium-labeled ISs, which exhibit extensive matrix effects, have been shown to be less accurate than matrix effect–free assays, which do not have isotopically labeled ISs.[40]

MATRIX CONSIDERATIONS FOR CALIBRATORS AND QUALITY CONTROLS

The composition of matrix for calibration curves in an LC-MS/MS assay may prove to be both consequential and irrelevant.[41] It may be consequential in that endogenous protein binding may play a significant role in the extraction efficiency of a procedure. It may be irrelevant in that the analytical performance is identical between the matrix of interest and water. As every test is different, hard and fast rules do not exist, but there are a few factors that should be considered when choosing calibration matrix.

First, charcoal-stripped matrix is a popular mechanism to provide surrogate matrix free of certain analytes. It should be recognized, however, that stripping of matrix fundamentally modifies the matrix, so "matrix-matched" is no longer a legitimate term.[42–44] Some matrices are stripped a number of times to remove endogenous background levels, further decreasing the actual matrix content. In the absence of a particular need for matrix constituents, such as albumin to act as a nonspecific binding partner in prevention of adsorptive loss, neat solvents may suffice. Alternatively, addition of additives, such as bovine serum albumin to neat solvents, can simplify calibration matrix preparation.[45,46]

If the matrix is then different from that of patient samples, questions of commutability of the assay's accuracy and precision claims between stripped matrix and authentic matrix rightly arise. In method development, adoption of experiments to address such questions early on should be performed. Important variables, such as protein binding of the spiked internal standard (specific or nonspecific) or ionization modifications due to endogenous components are experimentally determinable events. Time course mixing studies with IS to reach equilibrium in binding and IS recovery during sample analysis in prevalidation, respectively, may be able to evaluate those variables. Equivalency of various matrices should be shown in method development early on by analysis of mixtures of the matrix types in known ratios.[47] Additionally, consistent monitoring of the transition ratios and performing extended chromatographic separations in the development process will help to reveal possible errors.

MATERIAL PURCHASE

Methods developed by a laboratory should be compared with external assays for the same compound, either by proficiency testing or alternative schemes for adjudicating interlaboratory agreement. Assays may perform in a similar fashion, exhibiting equivalent matrix effects, recovery, and so forth, yet yield different results. This may be due to the selection of calibration material. The source material for calibration is of utmost importance in determining the accuracy of an analytical method; it is the primary factor by which all results are generated. To ensure harmonization (and thus agreement with peer groups in analysis of specimens), it is recommended that the compound(s) to be analyzed are sourced from more than one manufacturer. Additionally, certificates of analysis or other proof of purity should be reviewed extensively in method development and should be based on recognized techniques for determining purity.[48]

With multiple preparations of the compound in hand, the laboratory can then evaluate the agreement of those materials with equivalent weighings, dilutions, and comparisons. Such data may prove to be highly informative, as shown in the evaluation of metanephrines between 2 distinct sources.[49] The report demonstrates the importance of both multiple sources of calibration material, but also the use of higher-order methods to evaluate material purity. Unfortunately, few analytes assayed via MS have well-established higher-order materials or methods.[50] Thus, the distribution of both calibration standards and human specimens to other laboratories during method development to evaluate the assay's general interlaboratory agreement is appropriate.

SUMMARY

The process of method development should establish a preliminary procedure that can be evaluated for prevalidation experiments. Such experiments should be used to gauge success of the assay before validation occurs by stressing the considerations normally ascribed to new methods as well as the considerations described in this article as recommended in guidance documents.[51] Stringent review of results from prevalidation should be performed such that possible errors are deduced and are addressed before validation and assay launch. Data appraisal should include transition ratio assessments, retention time consistency, peak shape (width and asymmetry measures), fluctuations in baseline noise, precision, ion suppression, and so forth. Use of isotopically labeled ISs allows for deduction of assay characteristics in the presence of matrix constituents, which is a unique feature of MS. Observed errors in final method development/prevalidation batches will yield a return to method development for correction.

REFERENCES

1. Leinenbach A, Pannee J, Dülffer T, et al. Mass spectrometry–based candidate reference measurement procedure for quantification of amyloid-β in cerebrospinal fluid. Clin Chem 2014;60:987–94.
2. Fanelli D. Negative results are disappearing from most disciplines and countries. Scientometrics 2012;90:891–904.
3. Kushnir MM, Rockwood AL, Nelson GJ, et al. Assessing analytical specificity in quantitative analysis using tandem mass spectrometry. Clin Biochem 2005;38: 319–27.
4. Rappold BA. Mass spectrometry selectivity, specifically. Clin Chem 2016;62: 54–156.
5. Kebarle P, Peschke M. On the mechanisms by which the charged droplets produced by electrospray lead to gas phase ions. Anal Chim Acta 2000;406:11–35.
6. Hewavitharana AK, Herath HMDR, Shaw PN, et al. Effect of solvent and electrospray mass spectrometer parameters on the charge state distribution of peptides–a case study using liquid chromatography/mass spectrometry method development for beta-endorphin assay. Rapid Commun Mass Spectrom 2010;24: 3510–4.
7. Cole RB. Some tenets pertaining to electrospray ionization mass spectrometry. J Mass Spectrom 2000;35:763–72.
8. Kiontke A, Oliveira-Birkmeier A, Opitz A, et al. Electrospray ionization efficiency is dependent on different molecular descriptors with respect to solvent pH and instrumental configuration. PLoS One 2016;11(12):e0167502.
9. Page JS, Kelly RT, Tang K, et al. Ionization and transmission efficiency in an electrospray ionization–mass spectrometry interface. J Am Soc Mass Spectrom 2007; 18:1582–90.

10. Grant R, Rappold BR. Development and validation of small molecule analytes by liquid chromatography-tandem mass spectrometry. In: Rifai N, Horvath AR, Wittwer C, editors. Tietz textbook of clinical chemistry and molecular diagnostics. St. Louis MO Elsevier; 2018. p. 326.
11. Annesley TM. Methanol-associated matrix effects in electrospray ionization tandem mass spectrometry. Clin Chem 2007;53:1827–34.
12. Lickteig A, Salske M, Rappold BA. Design of optimization: how to improve performance of high-volume clinical LC/MS/MS assays; Proceedings of the 63rd ASMS Conference on Mass Spectrometry and Allied Topics, St Louis MO, May 31-June 4, 2015. [abstract: MP326].
13. Napoli KL. More on methanol-associated matrix effects in electrospray ionization mass spectrometry. Clin Chem 2009;55:1250–2.
14. Bristow AW, Nichols WF, Webb KS, et al. Evaluation of protocols for reproducible electrospray in-source collisionally induced dissociation on various liquid chromatography/mass spectrometry instruments and the development of spectral libraries. Rapid Commun Mass Spectrom 2002;16:2374–86.
15. Little JL, Williams AJ, Pshenichnov A, et al. Identification of known unknowns utilizing accurate mass data and ChemSpider. J Am Soc Mass Spectrom 2012;23:179–85.
16. Bennett PK, Van Horne KC. Identification of the major endogenous and persistent compounds in plasma, serum, and tissue that cause matrix effects with electrospray LC/MS techniques. American Association of Pharmaceutical Scientists Conference, Salt Lake City, Utah, Oct 24-25 2003.
17. Little JL, Wempe MF, Buchanan CM. Liquid chromatography–mass spectrometry/mass spectrometry method development for drug metabolism studies: examining lipid matrix ionization effects in plasma. J Chromatogr B Analyt Technol Biomed Life Sci 2006;833:219–30.
18. Rappold BA, Grant RP. HILIC-MS/MS method development for targeted quantitation of metabolites: practical considerations from a clinical diagnostic perspective. J Sep Sci 2011;34:3527–37.
19. Hammerling JA. A review of medical errors in laboratory diagnostics and where we are today. Lab Med 2015;43:41–4.
20. Wallace AM, Gibson SI, De La Hunty A, et al. Measurement of 25-hydroxyvitamin D in the clinical laboratory: current procedures, performance characteristics and limitations. Steroids 2010;75:477–88.
21. Stout PR, Horn CK, Lesser DR. Loss of THCCOOH from urine specimens stored in polypropylene and polyethylene containers at different temperatures. J Anal Toxicol 2000;247:567–71.
22. Grant R, Rappold B. Development and validation of quantitative LC-MS/MS assays for use in clinical diagnostics, mass spectrometry applications to the clinical laboratory Conference, Renaissance Hotel & Palm Springs Convention Center, Palm Springs CA, 2015, 2016, 2017, short course.
23. Zhang L, Henion J. LC/MS/MS bioanalytical protocol for determining the degree of non-specific binding in multi-well plates, Proceedings of the 65th/ASMS Conference on Mass Spectrometry and Allied Topics, Indianapolis, IN, June 4–8, 2017.
24. Wells D. Sample preparation for mass spectrometry applications. In: Rifai N, Horvath AR, Wittwer C, editors. Tietz textbook of clinical chemistry and molecular diagnostics. St. Louis MO Elsevier; 2018. p. 324.
25. Chambers E, Wagrowski-Diehl DM, Lu Z, et al. Systematic and comprehensive strategy for reducing matrix effects in LC/MS/MS analyses. J Chromatogr B Analyt Technol Biomed Life Sci 2007;852:22–34.

26. Polson C, Sarkar P, Incledon B, et al. Optimization of protein precipitation based upon effectiveness of protein removal and ionization effect in liquid chromatography–tandem mass spectrometry. J Chromatogr B Analyt Technol Biomed Life Sci 2003;785:263–75.

27. Marney LC, Laha TJ, Baird GS, et al. Isopropanol protein precipitation for the analysis of plasma free metanephrines by liquid chromatography–tandem mass spectrometry. Clin Chem 2008;54:1729–32.

28. Grant RP. Design and utility of open-access liquid chromatography tandem mass spectrometry in quantitative clinical toxicology and therapeutic drug monitoring. Trends Analyt Chem 2016;84:51–60.

29. Taylor PJ. Matrix effects: the Achilles heel of quantitative high-performance liquid chromatography–electrospray–tandem mass spectrometry. Clin Biochem 2005; 38:328–34.

30. Bonfiglio R, King RC, Olah TV, et al. The effects of sample preparation methods on the variability of the electrospray ionization response for model drug compounds. Rapid Commun Mass Spectrom 1999;30:1175–85.

31. Dams R, Huestis MA, Lambert WE, et al. Matrix effect in bio-analysis of illicit drugs with LC-MS/MS: influence of ionization type, sample preparation, and biofluid. J Am Soc Mass Spectrom 2003;14:1290–4.

32. Santa T. Derivatization reagents in liquid chromatography/electrospray ionization tandem mass spectrometry. Biomed Chromatogr 2011;25:1–10.

33. Iwasaki Y, Nakano Y, Mochizuki K, et al. A new strategy for ionization enhancement by derivatization for mass spectrometry. J Chromatogr B Analyt Technol Biomed Life Sci 2011;879:1159–65.

34. Held PK, White L, Pasquali M. Quantitative urine amino acid analysis using liquid chromatography tandem mass spectrometry and aTRAQ® reagents. J Chromatogr B Analyt Technol Biomed Life Sci 2011;879:2695–703.

35. Van Eeckhaut A, Lanckmans K, Sarre S, et al. Validation of bioanalytical LC–MS/MS assays: evaluation of matrix effects. J Chromatogr B Analyt Technol Biomed Life Sci 2009;877:2198–207.

36. Chavez-Eng CM, Constanzer ML, Matuszewski BK. High-performance liquid chromatographic-tandem mass spectrometric evaluation and determination of stable isotope labeled analogues of rofecoxib in human plasma samples from oral bioavailability studies. J Chromatogr B Analyt Technol Biomed Life Sci 2002;767:117–29.

37. Shuford CM, Sederoff RR, Chiang VL, et al. Peptide production and decay rates affect the quantitative accuracy of protein cleavage isotope dilution mass spectrometry (PC-IDMS). Mol Cell Proteomics 2012;11:814–23.

38. Jemal M, Schuster A, Whigan DB. Liquid chromatography/tandem mass spectrometry methods for quantitation of mevalonic acid in human plasma and urine: method validation, demonstration of using a surrogate analyte, and demonstration of unacceptable matrix effect in spite of use of a stable isotope analog internal standard. Rapid Commun Mass Spectrom 2003;17: 1723–34.

39. Wang S, Cyronak M, Yang E. Does a stable isotopically labeled internal standard always correct analyte response? A matrix effect study on a LC/MS/MS method for the determination of carvedilol enantiomers in human plasma. J Pharm Biomed Anal 2007;43:701–7.

40. Sancho JV, Pozo OJ, López FJ, et al. Different quantitation approaches for xenobiotics in human urine samples by liquid chromatography/electrospray tandem mass spectrometry. Rapid Commun Mass Spectrom 2002;16:639–45.

41. Hewavitharana AK. Matrix matching in liquid chromatography–mass spectrometry with stable isotope labelled internal standards—is it necessary? J Chrom A 2011;1218:359–61.

42. Cao Z, West C, Norton-Wenzel CS, et al. Effects of resin or charcoal treatment on fetal bovine serum and bovine calf serum. Endocr Res 2009;34:101–8.

43. Dang ZC, Lowik CWGM. Removal of serum factors by charcoal treatment promotes adipogenesis via a MAPK-dependent pathway. Mol Cell Biochem 2005; 268:159–67.

44. Sikora MJ, Johnson MD, Lee AV, et al. Endocrine response phenotypes are altered by charcoal-stripped serum variability. Endocrinology 2016;157:3760–6.

45. Strathmann FG, Laha TJ, Hoofnagle AN. Quantification of 1α, 25-dihydroxy vitamin D by immunoextraction and liquid chromatography–tandem mass spectrometry. Clin Chem 2011;57:1279–85.

46. Minkler PE, Stoll MS, Ingalls ST, et al. Quantification of carnitine and acylcarnitines in biological matrices by HPLC electrospray ionization–mass spectrometry. Clin Chem 2008;54:1451–62.

47. Clinical and Laboratory Standards Institute. Interference testing in clinical chemistry; approved guideline—second edition. CLSI document EP7–A2. Wayne (PA): Clinical and Laboratory Standards Institute; 2005.

48. Duewer DL, Parris RM, White E, et al. An approach to the metrologically sound traceable assessment of the chemical purity of organic reference materials. No. Special Publication (NIST SP)-1012. National Institute of Standards and Technology, Gaithersburg (MD): 2004.

49. Singh RJ, Grebe SK, Yue B, et al. Precisely wrong? Urinary fractionated metanephrines and peer-based laboratory proficiency testing. Clin Chem 2005;51: 472–4.

50. IFCC reference materials list. Available at: http://www.ifcc.org/ifcc-scientific-division/reference-materials/. Accessed January 10, 2018.

51. CLSI. Liquid chromatography-mass spectrometry methods; approved guideline. CLSI document C62-A. Wayne (PA): Clinical and Laboratory Standards Institute; 2014.

Development of a 25-Hydroxyvitamin D Liquid Chromatography–Tandem Mass Spectrometry Assay, Cleared by the Food and Drug Administration, via the De Novo Pathway

Nicole V. Tolan, PhD, DABCC[a,b],*

KEYWORDS

- FDA de novo pathway • Traceable LC-MS/MS method
- CDC Vitamin D Standardization Certification Program (VDSCP)
- 25-Hydroxyvitamin D2 • 3-Epi-25-hydroxyvitamin D

KEY POINTS

- The US Food and Drug Administration (FDA) has supported in vitro diagnostic device manufacturers by holding key public meetings and workshops, including mock 510(k) pre-submission document guidance.
- With a number of Clinical and Laboratory Standards Institute documents focusing specifically on mass spectrometry, manufacturers have guidance for each area of the verification studies necessary for FDA submission.
- Submitting a more accurate, traceable LC-MS/MS method that outperforms and is not substantially equivalent to predicate immunoassay methods requires following the *de novo* pathway; a more costly endeavor.
- Without a more rapid and less costly FDA review process, clinical laboratories must either send specific samples out to a commercial laboratory running a mass spectrometry-based method or develop their own laboratory developed tests (LDTs).

Continued

Disclosure Statement: Employment or leadership: SCIEX. Consultant or advisory role: None declared. Stock ownership: None declared. Honoraria: None declared. Research funding: SCIEX provided materials and reagents for the cited study. Expert testimony: None declared. Role of Sponsor: The sponsor, SCIEX, (a) conducted final FDA studies and (b) reviewed and approved the final article.
[a] Department of Anatomic and Clinical Pathology, Tufts University School of Medicine, 800 Washington Street, Boston, MA 02111, USA; [b] SCIEX Diagnostics, 500 Old Connecticut Path, Framingham, MA 01701, USA
* SCIEX, 500 Old Connecticut Path, Framingham, MA 01701.
E-mail address: nicole.tolan@sciex.com

Clin Lab Med 38 (2018) 553–564
https://doi.org/10.1016/j.cll.2018.05.006
0272-2712/18/© 2018 Elsevier Inc. All rights reserved.

labmed.theclinics.com

BACKGROUND

Vitamin D plays an essential role as a hormone in the control of calcium homeostasis and maintaining overall bone health.[1,2] Vitamin D and its metabolites are fat-soluble secosteroids, named for the broken carbon ring (Latin *secare*—to cut) as they are formed from provitamins D_3 and D_2 (**Fig. 1**). Both vitamin D_3 (cholecalciferol) and vitamin D_2 (ergocalciferol) are available as over-the-counter (non-prescription) supplements. Vitamin D_3 is found in few naturally occurring dietary sources, such as fish liver oils, fatty fish, egg yolks, and liver, but is also produced endogenously by exposure to sunlight, or

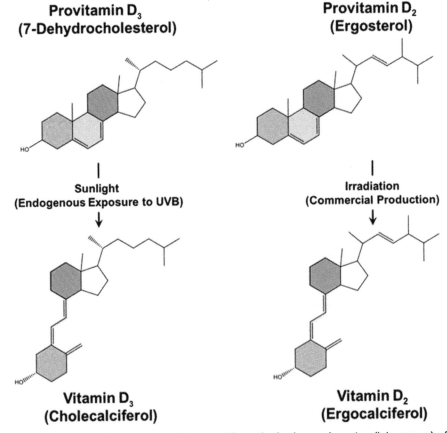

Fig. 1. Production of the secosteroids named from the broken carbon ring (lain: *secare*) of their provitamin D forms. Vitamin D_3 (cholecalciferol) is produced via sunlight, endogenous exposure to ultraviolet B radiation, and vitamin D_2 (ergocalciferol) from irradiation of yeast in commercial production.

ultraviolet B radiation, through the skin. Vitamin D_2 is produced by irradiation of yeast and is only made biologically available through direct vitamin supplementation and dietary intake.[3] It is generally accepted that individuals in the northern hemisphere do not have sufficient exposure to sunlight to maintain adequate levels of vitamin D. As a result, foods such as cereals, bread products, and milk are commonly fortified with vitamin D_3 or vitamin D_2. Despite this fortification and the ability to endogenously produce vitamin D_3 through sun exposure, general population supplementation has been recommended by the Institute of Medicine[4] to support overall bone health.

Both vitamin D_3 and D_2 are metabolized to 25-hydroxyvitamin D_3 (25(OH)D_3) and 25-hydroxyvitamin D_2 (25(OH)D_2), respectively, by 24-hydroxylase (CYP24A1) produced in the liver (**Fig. 2**). The conversion of 25(OH)D_3 and D_2 to the biologically active forms, 1,25-dihydroxyvitamin D_3 (1,25(OH2)D_3) and 1,25-dihydroxyvitamin D_2 (1,25(OH2)D_2), respectively, is regulated by 1α-hydroxylase in response to parathyroid hormone (PTH) concentrations. This process , in turn, increases calcium absorption through the intestine and, to a lesser extent, activates osteoclast activity to mobilize minerals, such as calcium, and digest the organic bone matrix, releasing alkaline phosphatase (ALP). This mechanism tightly regulates the concentration of circulating calcium via the calcium receptors of PTH, producing a negative feedback to downregulate PTH secretion with sufficient free calcium concentrations (**Fig. 3**). The concentration of 25(OH)D is best interpreted with other laboratory results, such as PTH levels, calcium (total, corrected by albumin when necessary), and phosphate.[5] Studies have shown that PTH decreases into the normal range with sufficient levels of 25(OH)D.[6] Elevated ALP can indicate increased bone turnover due to increased osteoclast activity in an effort to maintain adequate circulating calcium concentrations.

The typical concentrations of 25(OH)D range from 10 to 50 ng/mL with a half-life of approximately 2 to 3 weeks, making it the best marker for determining and monitoring a patient's overall vitamin D status. The biologically active form, 1,25(OH2)D, has a shorter half-life of around 4 to 6 hours and is much lower in concentration, approximately 0.01 to 0.05 ng/mL.[3] Direct measurement of 1,25(OH2)D is only recommended

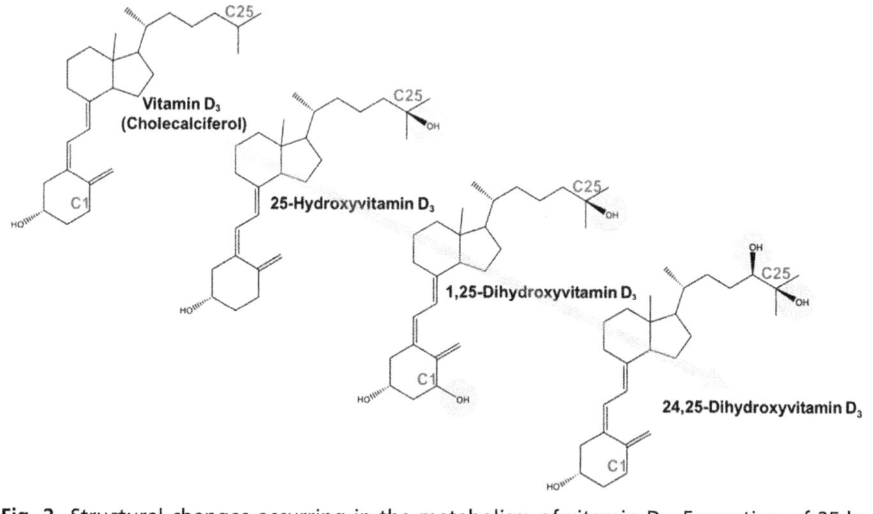

Fig. 2. Structural changes occurring in the metabolism of vitamin D_3. Formation of 25-hydroxyvtiamin D occurs via 24-hydroxylase (CYP24A1) produced in the liver, the biologically active form 1,25-dihydroxyvitamin D is converted via 1α-hydroxylase in the kidney, and its catabolism to 24,24-dihydroxyvitamin D_3 occurs before excretion.

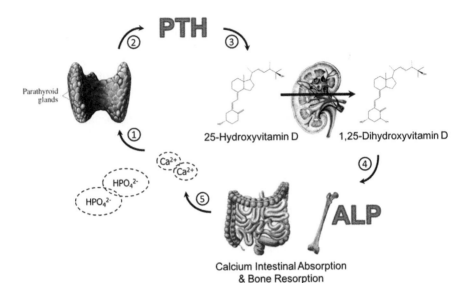

Fig. 3. Regulation of circulating calcium concentrations via negative feedback to the parathyroid glands. With reduced concentrations of free, ionized calcium, the parathyroid will increase circulating concentrations of parathyroid hormone (PTH), which will in turn increase the production of 1,25-dihydroxyvitamin D. This, the biologically active form, then acts principally in the intestines to increase calcium absorption and stimulates bone remodeling, which increases serum alkaline phosphatase (ALP) concentrations as well as circulating calcium. Adequate free calcium then provides negative feedback to the parathyroid to maintain PTH concentrations within the normal range.

in the investigation of a limited number of clinical conditions, such as granulomatous disease (increased), hyperparathyroidism (increased), hypercalcemia of malignancy, and in the rare case of differentiation of type I (synthesis defect) and type II (receptor defect) rickets.[2,5] It is also important to note that the concentration of 1,25(OH2)D is more variable due to its biologically active role. Precise measurement of this metabolite is currently limited to laboratory-developed tests (LDTs) using high-sensitivity mass spectrometry instruments.

Despite previous risk association studies suggesting the role of vitamin D in various conditions ranging from hypertension and cardiovascular disease to cancer and overall mortality,[5,7] no national primary care professional organization currently recommends population-wide screening for vitamin D. This was intentionally "insufficiency/deficiency" because of the divergent reference intervals recommended by the Institute of Medicine and the Endocrinology Society Guidelines. However, there are a number of clinical conditions where vitamin D status should be monitored via the measurement of 25(OH)D[8]:

- Patients with clinical symptoms or presentation of poor bone health (rickets, osteopenia/porosis, osteomalacia, or history of non-traumatic fractures);
- Increased metabolism and catabolism of 25(OH)D (primary hyperparathyroidism or hypercalcemia of malignancy);
- Malabsorption syndromes (inflammatory bowel disease, Crohn's disease, bariatric surgery);
- Decreased production of 25(OH)D (liver disease or hepatic failure);
- Altered production of 1,25(OH2)D (kidney disease, granulomatous disease); and
- Patients taking medications known to increase the risk of poor musculoskeletal health (antiseizure medications, glucocorticoids or HIV/AIDS medications).

METHODS FOR THE MEASUREMENT OF 25-HYDROXYVITAMIN D

Currently, the two most common methods for the determination of circulating concentrations of 25(OH)D are immunoassay and liquid chromatography tandem mass spectrometry (LC-MS/MS). In LC-MS/MS methods, the two forms of $25(OH)D_3$ and D_2 must also be reported as total 25(OH)D to provide clinicians with a clear assessment of overall vitamin D stores. Many laboratories are currently using the throughput advantages of high-volume automated immunoassay analyzers for the determination of 25(OH)D, because the volume of testing has exponentially increased with the introduction of increased risk associations with hypovitaminosis D in the lay literature.[7] Since the early 2000s, clinical laboratories have seen a dramatic increase (5- to 6-fold) in 25(OH)D testing,[9] which represented an 83-fold increase in reimbursement volume from 2000 to 2010 in Medicare Part B payments.[10]

Although commonly thought to only exist in the pediatric population, studies have shown that there is a significant concentration of the biologically inactive 3-epi-25-hydroxyvitamin D (3-epi-25(OH)D) forms found in adult serum, because the concentration is proportional to that of 25(OH)D.[11,12] Additionally, studies have demonstrated increased ionization efficiency of the 3-epimer forms, which in the absence of chromatographic resolution, increases the potential for interference even beyond their circulating concentrations.[13] Despite recent reports of high-throughput methods, the vast majority of LC-MS/MS LDTs used in clinical laboratories do not resolve the 3-epimer interferents from $25(OH)D_3$ and D_2.[14] Conversely, a Vitamin D External Quality Assessment Scheme (DEQAS) proficiency testing survey has confirmed that the widely used immunoassays are not subject to interferences from these isobaric compounds.[15] However, the immunoassay methods available today continue to suffer from poor recoveries of $25(OH)D_2$[16–18] and, until recently, the only form of high-dose vitamin D (50,000 IU) in the US has been that of vitamin D_2. Even with great improvement in 25(OH)D assay standardization and decreased interlaboratory imprecision across methods under the Center for Disease Control and Prevention's (CDC) Vitamin D Standardization Program (VDSCP), with the development of reference measurement procedures (RMPs),[15,19,20] poor recoveries of $25(OH)D_2$ remain. Unfortunately, of the standard reference materials (SRM) available through National Institute of Standards and Technology (NIST) and the CDC, only ten contain detecpaint concentrations of $25(OH)D_2$ and, of these, only a single SRM (NIST SRM 972a, level 3 = 13.3 ng/mL) contains a sufficient concentration to test the performance of commercially available immunoassays and LC-MS/MS LDTs.

Recently, we have evaluated the accuracy of three immunoassay methods against the first CDC/NIST-traceable, CDC VDSCP Vitamin D 200M Topaz™ LC-MS/MS method (SCIEX, Framingham, MA) cleared by the US Food and Drug Administration (FDA).[21] Supported by adequate performance on recent DEQAS and College of American Pathologists Accuracy-Based Vitamin D (ABVD). Proficiency testing surveys, we assumed complete recovery (100%) of $25(OH)D_3$ and determined the percent cross-recovery for $25(OH)D_2$ to be significantly lower than that specified in the package inserts for three immunoassay methods. We determined that patients with $25(OH)D_2$ concentrations greater than 20 ng/mL had mean recoveries ranging from 5.6 to −20.3 ng/mL different than the CDC-traceable SCIEX reference method (**Fig. 4**). Further, through random sampling, we observed that more than 8% of our vitamin D testing volume (37,500 samples per year) had concentrations greater than 20 ng/mL $25(OH)D_2$, and we conservatively estimated that 3000 samples would have inaccurate results annually, not an insignificant number being clinically discordant. Unfortunately, because immunoassays only provide total 25(OH)D concentrations, it is not possible to

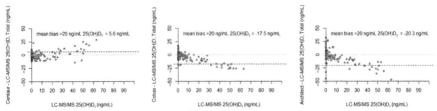

Fig. 4. Bland-Altman difference plots shown as a function of 25-hydroxyvitmain D_2 concentration, as determined by liquid chromatography tandem mass spectrometry (LC-MS/MS). The mean biases in total 25-hydroxyvitamin D for each immunoassay and the reference LC-MS/MS method in those samples containing >20 ng/mL 25-hydroxyvitamin D_2 are shown as dashed gray lines. The differences are demonstrated to be proportional to the under- or over-recovery of 25-hydroxyvitamin D_2 by the immunoassay methods and range from 5.6 to -20.3 ng/mL. (*Data from* Tolan NV, Yoon EJ, Brady AR, et al. Price of high-throughput 25-Hydroxyvitamin D Immunoassays: frequency of inaccurate results. JALM 2017;2;6:868–79; with permission.)

differentiate which samples would require additional LC-MS/MS confirmation testing to accurately quantitate the 25(OH)D_2 contribution to total vitamin D stores.

The clinical consequences of inaccurate 25(OH)D determination is relatively benign; however, under-recovery may lead to unnecessary diagnostic testing and clinical work-up for malabsorption or other clinical conditions. Inaccurate recoveries could contribute to false assessment of vitamin D stores in patients receiving high-dose supplementation where prolonged treatment could potentially lead to downstream clinical sequelae of hypervitaminosis D. Conversely, improved accuracy was obtained by the LC-MS/MS reference method due to improved analytical sensitivity and specificity.

THE NEED FOR MASS SPECTROMETRY-BASED METHODS IN CLINICAL LABORATORIES

From a historical perspective, mass spectrometry as a technology first began in the basic science research laboratories. Over the past 20 years, we have seen a dramatic increase in the number of scientific publications using the analytical technique of mass spectrometry, which occurred three times more frequently than the total number of articles published in 2014.[22] Expansion into the clinical laboratory has evolved from monitoring discrete small molecules to hundreds in a single injection, from small proteolytic peptides to intact proteins and their posttranslational modifications.

All experts would agree that, of the advances mass spectrometry has afforded the clinical laboratory, newborn screening has been the most impactful and rewarding.[23] From when Robert Guthrie developed the first blood test for phenylketonuria in 1961, to when in the 1980s Charles Roe, Steven Kahler, and David Millington developed newborn screening as we know it today, newborn screening received FDA clearance in 2008[24] and has saved thousands of lives worldwide. However, laboratorians face the dilemma of the lack of FDA-approved/cleared methods. For example, many clinical laboratories use the only FDA-cleared mass spectrometry-based method for tacrolimus,[25] but are modifying the method to also include cyclosporine, sirolimus, and everolimus to provide clinicians with accurate immunosuppressant quantitation and, because empirically, we know that physicians do sometimes order the wrong test (an advantage to multianalyte mass spectrometry panel assays).

In the absence of mass spectrometry, most laboratories perform immunoassays for the vast majority of testing and send samples out to a commercial laboratory when increased accuracy and precision are required (e.g., testosterone in women and children) or when immunoassay methods are incapable of producing accurate results (e.g., thyroglobulin in patients with detectable antithyroglobulin antibodies). Most often, a fast turnaround time is not seemingly necessary for these tests. However, considering the current health care environment, where physicians are expected to treat an increasing number of patients each day in an overly complicated structure with difficult medical record systems, a major focus has turned to gaining efficiencies in workflow with reduced staffing and realizing gains in reducing length of stay/readmit rates or unnecessary testing and clinical workup.

Mass spectrometry is now becoming increasingly automated with many of the same features and conveniences of today's high volume, automated analyzers. The SCIEX Vitamin D 200M assay for the Topaz LC-MS/MS system was designed to lower the barrier of adoption of mass spectrometry in routine clinical laboratories by providing FDA-cleared reagents (calibrators, controls, etc.) with a simplified operation (locked assay) and streamlined software. This offers the opportunity for clinical laboratories to provide higher quality results in house, faster, while commonly reducing costs or capturing lost revenue. In fact, many institutions are opting to run mass spectrometry-based methods in place of routine immunoassay methods, such as in direct-to-definitive pain management testing. As Dr Stacy Melanson points out, "it [doesn't] make sense to screen for something that 80% of the time will require confirmatory or definitive testing" and mass spectrometry offers the technical capacity to do so.[26]

US FOOD AND DRUG ADMINISTRATION SUBMISSION PROCESS

Many manufacturers face challenges when bringing new methods to market. The most scrutinized aspect of which is the need to demonstrate the performance of the method. In the premarket notification 510(k) process, the FDA currently relies on manufacturers to demonstrate substantial equivalence to an existing method. This is the principle pathway to obtain market authorization for most devices. However, this process is in contrast with ongoing accuracy-based standardization efforts. For example, Herold and Fitzgerald have demonstrated that all commercially available, FDA-cleared testosterone immunoassays provide inaccurate results in women and children as compared with the isotope dilution gas chromatography mass spectrometry reference method,[27] where the immunoassays were shown to be even less accurate than a random number generator. Bringing a new, traceable, accurate LC-MS/MS method to market that outperforms and is not substantially equivalent to current predicate methods would require following the de novo pathway, a more costly endeavor.

We experienced this first-hand when working with the FDA through our pre-market submissions for the SCIEX Vitamin D 200M assay. The FDA has stated that the mass spectrometry-based vitamin D assay raises different questions of safety and efficacy than the predicate immunoassays. Since the SCIEX method was developed with traceability to the CDC RMP through the NIST SRMs and incorporates protein precipitation and chromatographic resolution from isobaric interferences of 25(OH)D, we performed the method comparison to the CDC vitamin D RMP, maintain VDSCP certification, and obtained FDA clearance via the de novo pathway (as opposed to a predicate immunoassay method). The technology (with increased accuracy) raises fewer risk issues, which is why LC-MS/MS vitamin D assays will be down-classified by FDA to Class II exempt, while immunoassays will remain Class II 510(k).

The mass spectrometry community and manufacturers of mass spectrometry-based IVD assays play a role in how these assays are processed by the FDA. At the recent Mass Spectrometry: Applications to the Clinical Laboratory (2018 MSACL US) conference, Drs Jeffery, Humbard, and Haznadar of the FDA presented a very valuable, and interactive session titled *FDA Overview of the Process for Clearance and Approval of Mass Spectrometry-based In Vitro Devices.*[28] Here, they highlighted the ability for manufacturers to follow one of five methods in demonstrating substantial equivalence to a "legally marked device in the US," also known as a predicate that does not require pre-market approval. With Class II medical devices, posing moderate risk and requiring special controls, the de novo pathway relies on clinical truth (rather than a predicate device as the comparator) through a reference method or clinical diagnosis. However, in the absence of RMPs recognized by the FDA, and without substantial equivalence to a predicate method (commonly an immunoassay), manufacturers may be faced with following the Class III pre-market approval pathway. This process, to some extent, is the major barrier to bringing FDA-cleared/approved mass spectrometry-based assays to market.

Considering the fundamental capabilities of mass spectrometry, this instrumentation has the potential to not only provide more accurate laboratory results, but also to decrease the total cost of health care by providing data-rich multianalyte panels that better detect various clinical conditions. However, considering the current FDA and Centers for Medicare and Medicaid Services environment, successful clearance of such an assay is exceedingly difficult. These multianalyte mass spectrometry-based tests would commonly require following the de novo or pre-market approval application process and are commonly coded as proprietary laboratory analyses (PLA) or multianalyte assays with algorithmic analyses (MAAA). The reimbursement rate is largely uncertain in light of the Protecting Access to Medicare Act of 2014 and other US reimbursement challenges specific to these codes. In our own experience, the FDA had required reporting total 25(OH)D instead of D_3 and D2 independently, following the single-analyte reporting structure of the predicate immunoassay methods. However, most, if not all, mass spectrometry-based LDTs available in clinical laboratories provide discrete reporting of D_3, D_2, and total 25(OH)D concentrations. Although only incremental in the assessment of a patient's vitamin D status, reporting D_3 and D_2 concentrations in addition to total 25(OH)D allows for physicians to better interpret their patients' results, assessing their compliance given their form of supplementation. Multianalyte reporting also capitalizes on the improved capabilities of the mass spectrometry method.

Through the process of obtaining FDA clearance, we have learned that communication is key. The FDA has supported IVD manufacturers by holding key public meetings and workshops, and has specifically focused on particular areas of confusion through mock 510(k) presubmission documents.[29-31] The FDA is actively working to help manufacturers better understand how to submit an application when a predicate device does not exist or the predicate device is not substantially equivalent. In addition, with a number of Clinical Laboratory Standards Institute (CLSI) documents focusing specifically on mass spectrometry, manufacturers have guidance for each area of the verification studies necessary for FDA submission.[32-37] This process for SCIEX also required upgrading our quality management system to support the development and registration of IVD methods. For us, internal project management was also key in launching both the Topaz LC-MS/MS Class I medical device system and the FDA-cleared via the de novo pathway Vitamin D 200M assay.

Not dissimilar to the validation of an LDT, the process of FDA submission for the SCIEX Vitamin D 200M assay included the verification studies of precision (repeatability and reproducibility), linearity (analytical measuring range), upper and lower limit of the measuring interval (ULMI, LLMI), accuracy, interference testing, and establishing normal reference intervals. The determination of total 25(OH)D in human serum samples was performed using the Topaz LC-MS/MS System (SCIEX) and the FDA studies were performed at three clinical trial sites and over multiple reagent lots following the specific CLSI guidelines for each study.

The Vitamin D 200M Assay for the Topaz System is intended for in vitro diagnostic use in the quantitative determination of 25(OH)D through the measurement of 25(OH)D_3 and 25(OH)D_2 in human serum using LC-MS/MS technology by a trained laboratory professional in a clinical laboratory. The assay is intended for use with the Topaz System. The Vitamin D 200M Assay for the Topaz System is intended to be used in conjunction with other clinical or laboratory data to assist the clinician in making individual patient management decisions in an adult population in the assessment of vitamin D sufficiency. In this method, 100 μL of samples and standards undergo protein crash with the addition of 25 μL precipitation reagent and 200 μL deuterated internal standard (IS) solution. After vortexing to liberate the 25(OH)D from the binding protein, the samples are centrifuged at 1500×g for 5 minutes and the supernatant is transferred to an autosampler vial for analysis. For the LC-MS/MS determination of total 25(OH)D, addition of 25(OH)D_3 and 25(OH)D_2, 40 μL is then injected into a 50 μL sample loop prior to a 6.2-minute per injection gradient LC separation incorporating 2-dimensional chromatography with trap and analytical columns (SCIEX). Operating in positive ion mode, this method provides chromatographic resolution of 25(OH)D_2, 25(OH)D_3, 3-epi-25(OH)D_3, and 3-epi-25(OH)D_2. The concentrations of 25(OH)D_3 and 25(OH)D_2 in patient samples were determined by monitoring two precursor/product pairs by multiple reaction monitoring using the SCIEX ClearCore™ MD 1.1 software (SCIEX).

Precision was determined through a multisite evaluation study. At each of the three sites, 7 samples (~4–90 ng/mL) were assayed as 5 replicate extractions each day, over 5 days. The intraassay repeatability coefficient of variation (%CV) ranged from 2.7% to 6.3% (4.2–90.9 ng/mL) for 25(OH)D_3, 4.3% to 5.7% (4.5–91.0 ng/mL) for 25(OH)D2, and 2.9% to 3.8% (8.8–182 ng/mL) for total 25(OH)D. The interassay reproducibility was 3.3% to 5.0% for 25(OH)D_3, 6.8% to 10.3% for 25(OH)D_2, and 4.2% to 6.1% for total 25(OH)D across these same concentration ranges.

Linearity studies were performed across multiple reagent lots, instruments, and operators. The linearity range was determined to be 2.0 to 200.0 ng/mL for 25(OH)D_3 and D_2, and 4.0 to 400.0 ng/mL for total 25(OH)D. Studies were also performed to establish the limit of quantitation (% bias and %CV of <20%) where six SRMs were run in replicates of five over five days. The limit of quantitation for 25(OH)D_3 and D_2 was determined to be 2.0 ng/mL and 1.5 ng/mL, respectively. The reportable range was determined from the linearity and limit of quantitation studies to be 2.0 to 160.0 ng/mL for 25(OH)D_3, 2.0 to 165.0 ng/mL 25(OH)D_2, and 4.0 to 325.0 ng/mL for total 25(OH)D.

Accuracy was evaluated by method comparison against the CDC and Ghent University Reference Method using 120 patient samples with concentrations from 5.6 to 154.0 ng/mL. Passing-Bablock linear regression of the method comparison for 120 real patient samples was described by the regression equation: $y = 0.96x - 0.35$ ($R^2 = 0.989$). In addition, this method has received VDSCP certification, which, along with special controls, supports continued traceability.

In total, 58 potential interferents including vitamin D analogs and metabolites, endogenous substances, as well as potential isobaric compounds or fragments were tested and no interferents were identified. Most notably, 3-epi-25(OH)D_3 and 3-epi-25(OH)D_2 interference is prevented through their chromatographic separation. Further, cross-talk between analytes and IS met the acceptability criteria and were demonstrated to be 3.4% and 0% at the LLMI and 0.8% and 0.6% at the ULMI for 25(OH)D_3 and 25(OH)D_2, respectively.

Although there are global reference intervals for 25(OH)D, established by the Institute of Medicine and the Endocrine Society, as part of the FDA submission we used non-parametric analysis of the 25(OH)D concentrations from 404 apparently healthy subjects to determine the reference interval. The study design excluded individuals who received more than 2000 IU/d supplementation, had a history of clinical conditions or medication known to affect the concentration of 25(OH)D, or had abnormal laboratory findings suggestive of altered calcium homeostasis. The subjects included 216 males (53.5%) and 188 females (46.5%) ranging in age from 21 to 75 years and were self-reported to be white (n = 234; 57.9%), black (n = 120; 29.7%), Asian (n = 19; 4.7%), and other/multiple races (n = 22; 5.5%). Samples were collected from consenting individuals residing in California, Florida, and Minnesota across 12 months. We determined the normal reference interval from these three distinct geographic regions to be 10.1 to 48.2 ng/mL for California, 8.6 to 48.3 ng/mL for Minnesota, and 9.1 to 49.0 for Florida. Interestingly, we did not observe significant differences in the central 95th percentiles of the reference intervals across the geographic locations where the samples were collected.

SUMMARY

Without a more rapid and less costly FDA-clearance process, clinical laboratory directors are faced with either sending particular tests/patient population samples out to a commercial laboratory or developing their own LDTs when the immunoassay methods are inadequate to support quality patient management.

The process of developing LDTs and brining in mass spectrometry is not yet as trivial of a technique to that of high-volume automated analyzers and requires specially trained staff.

It is important for us to emphasize that not all LC-MS/MS LDTs are equal. In the past, we have seen large recalls of clinical laboratory results due to the absence of RMPs, non-commutable SRMs, or the use of standards that are not traceable.

LDTs will always exist, as we identify new biomarkers and improve technology in the clinical laboratory. However, further increase in the costs and complexity of obtaining FDA clearance/approval will only prolong the need for clinical laboratories to run said LDTs. Working together, clinical laboratories, IVD manufacturers, and the FDA will need to continue to maintain the rigorous testing and quality processes necessary to ensure patient safety, but also reduce the barriers to expedite the entry of LC-MS/MS in clinical laboratories.

REFERENCES

1. Tolan NV. Vitamin D. In: Rifai N, editor. New England journal of medicine knowledge+ and American association for clinical chemistry learning lab adaptive learning program. 2017. Available at: https://prod.area9labs.com. Accessed July 12, 2017.
2. Risteli J, Winter W, Kleerekoper M, et al. In: Burtis CA, Ashwood ER, Bruns DA, editors. Tietz textbook of clinical chemistry and molecular diagnostics vol. 5th edition. St. Louis (MO): Saunders Elsevier; 2012. p. 1765.
3. McCudden C. Vitamin D. 2012. Available at: http://media.aacc.org/Shows/Pearls/McCuddenVitaminD3-5-12/player.html. Accessed July 12, 2017.
4. Ross AC, Taylor CL, Yaktine AL, Del Valle BH, editors. Dietary Reference Intakes for Calcium and Vitamin D Institute of Medicine (US) Committee to Review Dietary Reference Intakes for Vitamin D and Calcium. Washington (DC): National Academies Press (US); 2011.
5. Holick MF. The D-lemma: to screen or not to screen for 25-hydroxyvitamin D concentrations. Clin Chem 2010;56:729–31.

6. Thomas MK, Lloyd-Jones DM, Thadhani RI, et al. Hypovitaminosis D in medical inpatients. N Engl J Med 1998;338:777–83.

7. Kolata G. D is for Dilemma. Why are so many people popping vitamin D? The New York Times; 2017.

8. Holick MF, Binkley NC, Bischoff-Ferrari HA, et al. Evaluation, treatment, and prevention of vitamin D deficiency: an Endocrine Society clinical practice guideline. J Clin Endocrinol Metab 2011;96:1911–30.

9. Scott MG, Gronowski AM, Reid IR, et al. Vitamin D: the more we know, the less we know. Clin Chem 2015;61:462–5.

10. Shahangian S, Alspach TD, Astles JR, et al. Trends in laboratory test volumes for Medicare Part B reimbursements, 2000-2010. Arch Pathol Lab Med 2014;138:189–203.

11. Lensmeyer G, Poquette M, Wiebe D, et al. The C-3 epimer of 25-hydroxyvitamin D(3) is present in adult serum. J Clin Endocrinol Metab 2012;97:163–8.

12. Strathmann FG, Sadilkova K, Laha TJ, et al. 3-epi-25 hydroxyvitamin D concentrations are not correlated with age in a cohort of infants and adults. Clin Chim Acta 2012;413:203–6.

13. van den Ouweland JM, Beijers AM, van Daal H. Overestimation of 25-hydroxyvitamin D3 by increased ionisation efficiency of 3-epi-25-hydroxyvitamin D3 in LC-MS/MS methods not separating both metabolites as determined by an LC-MS/MS method for separate quantification of 25-hydroxyvitamin D3, 3-epi-25-hydroxyvitamin D3 and 25-hydroxyvitamin D2 in human serum. J Chromatogr B Analyt Technol Biomed Life Sci 2014;967:195–202.

14. Yang Y, Rogers K, Wardle R, et al. High-throughput measurement of 25-hydroxyvitamin D by LC-MS/MS with separation of the C3-epimer interference for pediatric populations. Clin Chim Acta 2016;454:102–6.

15. Carter GD. 25-hydroxyvitamin D: a difficult analyte. Clin Chem 2012;58:486–8.

16. Shu I, Pina-Oviedo S, Quiroga-Garza G, et al. Influence of vitamin D2 percentage on accuracy of 4 commercial total 25-hydroxyvitamin D assays. Clin Chem 2013;59:1273–5.

17. Le Goff C, Peeters S, Crine Y, et al. Evaluation of the cross-reactivity of 25-hydroxyvitamin D2 on seven commercial immunoassays on native samples. Clin Chem Lab Med 2012;50:2031–2.

18. Li L, Zeng Q, Yuan J, et al. Performance evaluation of two immunoassays for 25-hydroxyvitamin D. J Clin Biochem Nutr 2016;58:186–92.

19. National Institutes of Health, Office of Dietary Supplements. Vitamin D Initiative. Available at: https://ods.od.nih.gov/Research/vdsp.aspx. Accessed February, 2016.

20. Mineva EM, Schleicher RL, Chaudhary-Webb M, et al. A candidate reference measurement procedure for quantifying serum concentrations of 25-hydroxyvitamin D(3) and 25-hydroxyvitamin D(2) using isotope-dilution liquid chromatography-tandem mass spectrometry. Anal Bioanal Chem 2015;407:5615–24.

21. Tolan NV, Yoon EJ, Brady AR, et al. Price of High-Throughput 25-Hydroxyvitamin D Immunoassays: Frequency of Inaccurate Results. Journal of Applied Lab Med 2017;2:461–3.

22. Annesley TM, Cooks RG, Herold DA, et al. Clinical mass spectrometry-achieving prominence in laboratory medicine. Clin Chem 2016;62:1–3.

23. Landau M. An interview with David Millington. Clin Chem 2016;62:12–9.

24. Jones G, Prosser DE, Kaufmann M. 25-hydroxyvitamin D-24-hydroxylase (CYP24A1): its important role in the degradation of vitamin D. Arch Biochem Biophys 2012;523:9–18.

25. FDA 510(k) Submission: waters masstrak immunosuppressants kit. Available at: https://www.accessdata.fda.gov/cdrh_docs/pdf6/K063868.pdf. Accessed December, 2017.
26. Titus K. Mass spec up front for pain management testing: Interest growing in oral fluid testing as alternative to urine testing. 2016. Available at: http://www.captodayonline.com/mass-spec-front-pain-management-testing-interest-growing-oral-fluid-testing-alternative-urine-testing/. Accessed June, 2016.
27. Herold DA, Fitzgerald RL. Immunoassays for testosterone in women: better than a guess? Clin Chem 2003;49:1250–1.
28. FDA Overview of the process for clearance and approval of mass spectrometry-based in vitro diagnostic devices. Available at: https://www.msacl.org/documents/2018US/slides/MSACL2018US_FDA_Discussion_Group_slides.pdf. Accessed January 29, 2018.
29. Lathrop JT, Jeffery DA, Shea YR, et al. US Food and Drug Administration perspectives on clinical mass spectrometry. Clin Chem 2016;62:41–7.
30. U.S. Food and Drug Administration. Public workshop on mass spectrometry in the clinic: regulatory considerations surrounding validation of liquid chromatography-mass spectrometry Based Devices. 2016. Available at: https://www.fda.gov/downloads/MedicalDevices/NewsEvents/WorkshopsConferences/UCM496805.pdf. Accessed September, 2017.
31. Regnier FE, Skates SJ, Mesri M, et al. Protein-based multiplex assays: mock pre-submissions to the US Food and Drug Administration. Clin Chem 2010;56:165–71.
32. CLSI document EP05-A3 Evaluation of precision of quantitative measurement procedures; approved guideline. 3rd edition. Wayne (PA): Clinical Laboratory Standards Institute (CLSI); 2014.
33. CLSI document EP06-A Evaluation of the linearity of quantitative measurement procedures: a statistical approach; approved guideline. 1st edition. Wayne (PA): Clinical Laboratory Standards Institute (CLSI); 2003.
34. CLSI document EP17–A2 Evaluation of detection capability for clinical laboratory measurement procedures; approved guideline. 2nd edition. Wayne (PA): Clinical Laboratory Standards Institute (CLSI); 2012.
35. CLSI document EP07-A2 Interference testing in clinical chemistry; approved guideline. 2nd edition. Wayne (PA): Clinical Laboratory Standards Institute (CLSI); 2005.
36. CLSI document EP07–A2 Defining, establishing, and verifying reference intervals in the clinical laboratory; approved guideline. 3rd edition. Wayne (PA): Clinical Laboratory Standards Institute (CLSI); 2010.
37. CLSI document C62-A Liquid chromatography-mass spectrometry methods; approved guidelines. Wayne (PA): Clinical Laboratory Standards Institute; 2014.

Moving?

Make sure your subscription moves with you!

To notify us of your new address, find your **Clinics Account Number** (located on your mailing label above your name), and contact customer service at:

Email: journalscustomerservice-usa@elsevier.com

800-654-2452 (subscribers in the U.S. & Canada)
314-447-8871 (subscribers outside of the U.S. & Canada)

Fax number: 314-447-8029

Elsevier Health Sciences Division
Subscription Customer Service
3251 Riverport Lane
Maryland Heights, MO 63043